THE BRAIN INJURY REHABILITATION WORKBOOK

T0321015

Also Available

Memory Rehabilitation:
Integrating Theory and Practice
Barbara A. Wilson

The Brain Injury Rehabilitation Workbook

Edited by

Rachel Winson
Barbara A. Wilson
Andrew Bateman

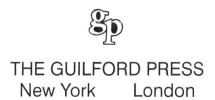

THE GUILFORD PRESS
New York   London

Copyright © 2017 The Guilford Press
A Division of Guilford Publications, Inc.
370 Seventh Avenue, Suite 1200, New York, NY 10001
www.guilford.com

All rights reserved

Except as noted, no part of this book may be reproduced, translated, stored in a retrieval system, or trans-
mitted, in any form or by any means, electronic, mechanical, photocopying, microfilming, recording, or
otherwise, without written permission from the publisher.

Printed in the United States of America

This book is printed on acid-free paper.

Last digit is print number: 9   8   7   6   5   4

The authors have checked with sources believed to be reliable in their efforts to provide information that is
complete and generally in accord with the standards of practice that are accepted at the time of publication.
However, in view of the possibility of human error or changes in behavioral, mental health, or medical sciences, neither the authors, nor the editors and publisher, nor any other party who has been involved in the
preparation or publication of this work warrants that the information contained herein is in every respect
accurate or complete, and they are not responsible for any errors or omissions or the results obtained from
the use of such information. Readers are encouraged to confirm the information contained in this book
with other sources.

LIMITED DUPLICATION LICENSE

These materials are intended for use only by qualified professionals.

The publisher grants to individual purchasers of this book nonassignable permission to reproduce all
materials for which permission is specifically granted in a footnote. This license is limited to you, the
individual purchaser, for personal use or use with individual clients. This license does not grant the right
to reproduce these materials for resale, redistribution, electronic display, or any other purposes (including but not limited to books, pamphlets, articles, video- or audiotapes, blogs, file-sharing sites, Internet
or intranet sites, and handouts or slides for lectures, workshops, or webinars, whether or not a fee is
charged). Permission to reproduce these materials for these and any other purposes must be obtained in
writing from the Permissions Department of Guilford Publications.

Library of Congress Cataloging-in-Publication Data

Names: Winson, Rachel, editor. | Wilson, Barbara A., 1941- editor. | Bateman,
    Andrew (Physical therapist) editor.
Title: The brain injury rehabilitation workbook / edited by Rachel Winson,
    Barbara A. Wilson, Andrew Bateman.
Description: New York : The Guilford Press, [2017] | Includes bibliographical
    references and index.
Identifiers: LCCN 2016035932 | ISBN 9781462528509 (paperback : alk. paper)
Subjects: | MESH: Brain Injuries—rehabilitation | Rehabilitation—methods
Classification: LCC RD594 | NLM WL 354 | DDC 617.4/810446—dc23
LC record available at *https://lccn.loc.gov/2016035932*

Illustrations by Lucy Driver.

About the Editors

Rachel Winson, MA, MSc, an advanced occupational therapist, is currently working as part of a community neurorehabilitation team at the University of East Anglia, in Norwich, Norfolk, United Kingdom. Previously, she worked at The Oliver Zangwill Centre for Neuropsychological Rehabilitation, in Ely, Cambridgeshire, United Kingdom, which provides high-quality evidence-based neuropsychological assessment and rehabilitation to patients with acquired brain injury. Ms. Winson has also worked in an acute inpatient stroke rehabilitation setting and in dementia research.

Barbara A. Wilson, OBE, PhD, a clinical neuropsychologist, is founder of The Oliver Zangwill Centre for Neuropsychological Rehabilitation. She has worked in brain injury rehabilitation since the 1970s. Dr. Wilson has published 23 books, 280 journal articles and book chapters, and 8 neuropsychological tests, and is editor of the journal *Neuropsychological Rehabilitation*. She has won many honors for her work, including three lifetime achievement awards, the Ramón y Cajal Award from the International Neuropsychiatric Association, and the M. B. Shapiro Award from the British Psychological Society. She is past president of the British Neuropsychological Society and the International Neuropsychological Society, and is currently president of the Encephalitis Society and on the management committee of the World Federation for NeuroRehabilitation. Dr. Wilson is a Fellow of the British Psychological Society, the Academy of Medical Sciences, and the Academy of Social Sciences. She is an honorary professor at the University of Hong Kong, the University of Sydney, and the University of East Anglia.

Andrew Bateman, PhD, a chartered physiotherapist, has been Clinical Manager at The Oliver Zangwill Centre since 2002. He has worked in research and clinical rehabilitation since 1990. Dr. Bateman has been involved in a range of research studies investigating patient-reported outcomes, executive functions, assistive technology, dyspraxia, and Rasch analysis.

Contributors

Andrew Bateman, PhD, The Oliver Zangwill Centre for Neuropsychological Rehabilitation, Ely, Cambridgeshire, United Kingdom

Susan Brentnall, DipCOT, The Oliver Zangwill Centre for Neuropsychological Rehabilitation, Ely, Cambridgeshire, United Kingdom

Jessica Fish, DClinPsy, The Oliver Zangwill Centre for Neuropsychological Rehabilitation, Ely, Cambridgeshire, United Kingdom

Catherine Longworth Ford, PhD, The Oliver Zangwill Centre for Neuropsychological Rehabilitation, Ely, Cambridgeshire, United Kingdom; Cambridgeshire Community Services National Health Service (NHS) Trust, St. Ives, Cambridgeshire, United Kingdom; Community Neuro-Rehabilitation, Cambridgeshire and Peterborough NHS Foundation Trust, Cambridge, Cambridgeshire, United Kingdom; and Health Education England, Leeds, West Yorkshire, United Kingdom

Fergus Gracey, DClinPsy, University of East Anglia, Norwich, Norfolk, United Kingdom; and Cambridgeshire Community Services NHS Trust, St. Ives, Cambridgeshire, United Kingdom

Emily Grader, BA, The Oliver Zangwill Centre for Neuropsychological Rehabilitation, Ely, Cambridgeshire, United Kingdom

Kathrin Hicks, DClinPsy, Cambridgeshire and Peterborough NHS Foundation Trust, Cambridge, Cambridgeshire, United Kingdom; Cambridge University Hospital NHS Trust, Cambridge, Cambridgeshire, United Kingdom

Clare Keohane, MRes, The Oliver Zangwill Centre for Neuropsychological Rehabilitation, Ely, Cambridgeshire, United Kingdom

Donna Malley, MSc, The Oliver Zangwill Centre for Neuropsychological Rehabilitation, Ely, Cambridgeshire, United Kingdom

Leyla Prince, MSc, The Oliver Zangwill Centre for Neuropsychological Rehabilitation, Ely, Cambridgeshire, United Kingdom

Barbara A. Wilson, OBE, PhD, The Oliver Zangwill Centre for Neuropsychological Rehabilitation, Ely, Cambridgeshire, United Kingdom; and The Raphael Medical Centre, Tonbridge, Kent, United Kingdom

Jill Winegardner, PhD, The Oliver Zangwill Centre for Neuropsychological Rehabilitation, Ely, Cambridgeshire, United Kingdom

Rachel Winson, MA, MSc, Cambridgeshire and Peterborough NHS Foundation Trust, Cambridge, Cambridgeshire, United Kingdom

Contents

Purchasers of this book can download and print the handouts
at *www.guilford.com/winson-forms* for personal use
or use with individual clients.

List of Handouts

CHAPTER 1

General Introduction

Barbara A. Wilson

"Neuropsychological rehabilitation" is a process whereby people who have sustained insults to the brain are helped to achieve their optimum physical, emotional, psychological, and vocational well-being (McLellan, 1991). The main purposes of such rehabilitation are to support people with disabilities resulting from brain insults in achieving their optimum level of well-being, to reduce the impact of their problems in everyday life, and to help them return to their own most appropriate environments. Rehabilitation is not about teaching clients to score better on tests, to learn lists of words, or to be faster at detecting stimuli. The focus of treatment is on improving aspects of everyday life; rehabilitation therefore needs to involve personally meaningful themes, activities, settings, and interactions (Ylvisaker & Feeney, 2000).

PRINCIPLES OF REHABILITATION

This workbook has grown out of the psychoeducation groups run for clients with acquired brain injury (ABI) who attend The Oliver Zangwill Centre (OZC) for Neuropsychological Rehabilitation in Ely, Cambridgeshire, United Kingdom. The rehabilitation program at OZC is based on six core components that the staff members believe illustrate the principles of good clinical practice, and that underpin the material offered in this book:

1. *Therapeutic milieu.* A concept derived from the work of Ben-Yishay (1996), the "therapeutic milieu" in holistic rehabilitation refers to the organization of all aspects of the environment to provide maximum support in the process of adjustment and increased social participation. The milieu embodies a strong sense of mutual cooperation and trust—a sense that underpins the working alliances between clients and clinicians.

2. *Meaningful goals.* Care is taken to make the goals set with clients meaningful and functionally relevant. By "meaningful functional activity," we are referring to all daily activities that form the basis for social participation. These can be categorized into vocational, educational, recreational, social, and independent living activities. It is through participation in these areas that we all gain a sense of purpose and meaning in our lives. Although we may not think about this consciously in everyday life, these types of activities enable us to achieve certain aims or ambitions that are personally significant to us and thereby contribute to our sense of identity.

3. *Shared understanding.* In a rehabilitation context, this term refers to mutual understanding among clients, families, and staff. The notion comes from the use of "formulation" in clinical practice (Butler, 1998). As explained in more detail below, a formulation is a map or guide to intervention that combines a model derived from established theories and best evidence from the client's and family's own personal views, experiences, and stories. This concept should be applied to all individual clinical work, and should influence the way the rehabilitation experience is organized as a whole. It includes a team philosophy that incorporates a shared team vision, explicit values, and goals. Additional characteristics of shared understanding include assimilation of research and theory; participation in knowledge and experience with other professionals and families; peer audit of the services provided; and absorption of the views and contributions of past clients.

4. *Psychological interventions.* These are based upon certain ways of understanding feelings and behavior. Specific psychological models are applied to guide work, depending upon each individual's specific needs. Approaches from these models provide ways for team members to engage clients in positive change and to tackle specific problems.

5. *Compensatory strategies and retraining.* These are the two principal approaches to managing cognitive impairments. "Compensatory strategies" are alternative ways to enable individuals to achieve a desired objective when an underlying function of the brain is not operating effectively; many of these are outlined in this workbook. "Retraining" is undertaken to improve performance of a specific brain function or to improve performance on a particular task or activity. Retraining also helps to address skills lost through lack of use (e.g., through not being at work since an injury occurred).

6. *Families and caregivers.* Rehabilitation involves working closely with families and caregivers, who sometimes report that they feel like "afterthoughts" in rehabilitation. Recent government policies within the United Kingdom highlight the fact that families and caregivers experience significant burden following ABI, and provision of support for them is recommended.

At OZC, we follow a holistic approach to brain injury rehabilitation, pioneered by Diller (1976), Ben-Yishay (1978), and Prigatano (1986). Such an approach "consists of well-integrated interventions that exceed in scope, as well as in kind, those highly specific and circumscribed interventions which are usually subsumed under the term 'cognitive remediation'" (Ben-Yishay & Prigatano, 1990, p. 400). Perhaps the main philosophy of the holistic approach is the insistence that it is futile to separate the cognitive, social, emotional, and functional aspects of brain injury. Given that emotions affect human behavior, including how people think, remember, communicate, and solve problems, we need to acknowledge that these functions are interconnected and often hard to separate; all of them need to be dealt with in rehabilitation.

Ben-Yishay and Prigatano (1990) provide a model of hierarchical stages in the holistic approach through which a client must work (either implicitly or explicitly) in rehabilitation:

- *Engagement:* Increasing the individual's awareness of what has happened to him or her.
- *Awareness:* Increasing the person's understanding of what has happened.
- *Mastery:* The provision of strategies or techniques to reduce cognitive problems.
- *Control:* The development of compensatory skills.
- *Acceptance.*
- *Identity:* Provision of vocational and other counseling.

It can be argued that the holistic approach is less of a model and more of a series of beliefs or principles (Prigatano, 1999). Nevertheless, the holistic model makes clinical sense—and in the long term it is probably cost-effective, despite its apparent expense (Cope, Cole, Hali, & Barkan, 1991; Mehlbye & Larsen, 1994; Wilson, 1997; Wilson & Evans, 2002).

In fact, there is mounting evidence that rehabilitation reduces the effects of cognitive, psychosocial, and emotional problems, leading to greater independence and eventual employability for many persons with brain injuries, as well as reductions in family stress (Cicerone et al., 2005; Wilson, Gracey, Evans, & Bateman, 2009). Cicerone, Mott, Azulay, Sharlow-Galella, Ellmo, et al. (2008) and Cicerone, Langenbahn, Braden, Malec, Berquist, et al. (2011) endorse the effectiveness of holistic approaches for traumatic brain injury (TBI): "Comprehensive holistic neuropsychological rehabilitation is recommended to improve post-acute participation and quality of life after moderate or severe TBI" (2011, p. 526).

Although the holistic approach is possibly best for the majority of people with brain injury, it is probably true to say that holistic programs can be improved through the incorporation of ideas and applications from learning theory, including task analysis, baseline recording, and monitoring. Other improvements can come from the implementation of single-case experimental designs within individual treatment programs. Further refinements can be encouraged by the use of cognitive neuropsychological models; such models enable us to identify cognitive strengths and weaknesses in more detail, to explain observed phenomena, and to make predictions about cognitive functioning.

THIS BOOK'S INTENDED AUDIENCE

While the myriad difficulties faced by survivors of brain injury—which can range from word-finding difficulties to memory problems to anger outbursts—require support from an experienced interdisciplinary team of speech and language therapists, occupational therapists, and clinical psychologists, few clients have such a team at their disposal. Many therapists and psychologists are working alone and may see clients at most on a weekly basis in a hospital or clinic. They may be seeing people at home, or they may be using Skype or other Internet-based methods of service provision, and they will probably not be working in a brain injury rehabilitation center. It is for these professionals that we have published this book. We envisage that it will be used primarily by occupational therapists, speech and language therapists, clinical psychologists, and neuropsychologists, as well as others working with survivors of TBI, stroke, encephalitis, hypoxic brain damage, and other kinds of nonprogressive brain injury. The workbook can be used in a hospital or clinic setting, but can also be used when therapists are visiting clients at home.

The resources provided in the book are aimed at supporting therapists' work across professional boundaries, using core skills to address clients' needs holistically. Please be aware that our intention is not to imply that occupational therapists can be clinical psychologists, or vice versa. It is important for professionals to be aware of their own disciplinary limitations, and to refer clients to appropriately qualified service providers when doing so is appropriate.

ISSUES IN REHABILITATION

Assessment

Before any treatment can begin, a careful assessment is necessary. Although Sundberg and Tyler (1962) best defined "assessment" over 50 years ago when they described the process as involving the systematic collection, organization, and interpretation of information about a person and his or her situation, assessment is also concerned with the prediction of behavior in new situations. The way this information is collected, organized, and interpreted will depend on the purpose of the assessment. Answering a theoretical question such as "Are there double dissociations between long-term and short-term memory deficits?" requires a particular approach to assessment. In this book, our aim is to help provide practical answers to practical questions, such as "How do the memory deficits manifest themselves in everyday life?"; this aim requires a completely different mode of assessment.

In clinical practice, there are two main types of assessment procedures: those where standardized assessment tools are employed, and those where more functional or behavioral measures are used. These distinctive types of assessment enable us to answer different questions. Standardized tests can tell us how a client compares to others of the same age or the same diagnosis. They can determine the cognitive strengths and weaknesses of the person being assessed; for instance, they can help us decide whether a client has a pure memory deficit or more widespread cognitive difficulties. They can also enable us to estimate the probability of clinical depression and so forth. Standardized assessment procedures, however, are less good at answering other questions important in rehabilitation, such as how the client's family is coping; what the client sees as his or her major problems; what compensatory strategies have been tried; whether this person is able to return home or return to work; or what learning strategies should be employed in teaching the client new information. These questions aim to understand practical problems the individual may face in real life. Ultimately, they are aimed at making daily living better for both the client and family. In another book, I (Wilson, 2009) provide further discussion of assessment and the characteristics of different kinds of assessment procedures; advice on assessment is also offered in each chapter of this book.

Formulation

When the assessment procedures have been completed, we can derive hypotheses regarding the nature, causes, and factors influencing a client's current situation and problems. In other words, we can come up with a "formulation." Formulation takes into account the multitude of possible influences on an individual's level of functioning and psychological state. It also helps the team, the individual therapist(s), and the client to understand the problems. In an interdisciplinary rehabilitation team, where a range of assessments (and interventions) may be carried out by different professionals, formulation helps bring together the results of these assessments into a single coherent whole. Included in the formulation should be a consideration of preinjury factors, such as the client's personality, occupation, and family support; the nature and type of injury, such as a life-threatening TBI; the extent of any losses, such as hemiplegia, memory impairment, and word-finding difficulties; and coping and adjustment issues. In the formulation process, cognitive, emotional, and behavioral consequences of the brain injury will be addressed, together with threats to identity and how the person makes sense of what has happened to him or her. Finally, the formulation should consider family and other social networks. Presenting this formulation visually, through a chart or graph, may help summarize the information and promote shared understanding (see Handout 1.1*).

A good clinical formulation should lead to appropriate and relevant interventions. We (Wilson, Robertson, & Mole, 2015) describe how formulation was used to set psychological therapy goals for Claire, who, following encephalitis, presented with anxiety symptoms that were formulated in terms of the threat to her identity. She had been a caring mother, wife, friend, and nurse. After the illness, however, she felt unable to run her household or take care of her children. Her anxiety symptoms further reduced her confidence in carrying out her household duties. Claire perceived a discrepancy between who she was before her illness and how she was defined after the illness. She had impairments in autobiographical memory and poor consolidation of new information. This, together with the perceived discrepancy, led her to do things to make herself feel "more like me" by the application of old, inflexible rules, and thus protect herself from this threat to her identity. The development of mood goals for her psychological therapy was based on this formulation.

Goal Setting

Goal setting has been used in rehabilitation for a number of years with various diagnostic groups, including people with cerebral palsy, spinal injuries, developmental learning difficulties, and ABI (McMillan & Sparkes, 1999). Because goal setting is simple, focuses on practical everyday problems, is tailored to individual needs, and avoids the artificial

---

*At the end of the chapter.

distinction between many outcome measures and real-life functioning, it is used increasingly in rehabilitation programs. Goal setting provides direction for rehabilitation, identifies priorities for intervention, evaluates progress, compartmentalizes treatment into achievable steps, promotes team functioning and cooperation, and results in better outcomes (Nair & Wade, 2003).

As mentioned above, it is important for rehabilitation to focus on the achievement of meaningful and functionally relevant goals. Levack et al. (2015) state, "There is general agreement that goal setting is a hallmark of contemporary rehabilitation and that skills in goal setting characterize those health professionals who work in this field" (p. 4). When we negotiate goals with our clients, their families, and the members of their rehabilitation teams, we are looking for something that the clients *will* do and *want* to do; these targets should reflect the clients' longer-term goals and be steps toward achieving them. Goals are important regulators and motivators of human performance and action (Austin & Vancouver, 1996); ultimately, they are a desired outcome by which progress can be measured.

From the earliest days of goal setting in brain injury rehabilitation (Houts & Scott, 1975; McMillan & Sparkes, 1999), several principles of this approach to rehabilitation have been recognized. First, each client should (as far as possible) be involved in setting his or her own goals. Second, the goals should be reasonable and client-centered. Third, they should describe the client's behavior when a goal is reached. Fourth, they should spell out the methods to be used in achieving the goals, in such a manner that anyone reading the plan would know what to do. McMillan and Sparkes (1999) summarize the principles of Houts and Scott (1975) and add to them by suggesting that goals should (1) be realistic and potentially attainable during admission, (2) be clear and specific, (3) have a definite time deadline, and (4) be measurable. These recommendations have been used to provide an acronym that reminds us that goals should be SMART (Specific, Measurable, Achievable, Realistic, and Timely; McMillan & Sparkes, 1999; Evans, 2012). Others have added an extra ER to make SMARTER goals, the last two letters referring (depending on the authors) to Evaluate and Revise (Yemm, 2013), Ethical and Recorded (Haughey, 2011), or Evolving and Relation-centered (Sherratt, Worrall, Hersh, Howe, & Davidson, 2015).

Kersten, McPherson, Kayes, Theadom, and McCambridge (2015) suggest some limitations of the SMART approach, but the main point is that the goals set for individuals in brain injury rehabilitation programs should be meaningful and purposeful for those individuals.

Long-term goals target disabilities in order to improve day-to-day functioning and should be achievable by the time of discharge from a rehabilitation program, whereas *short-term goals* are the steps set each week or two to achieve the long-term goals. Collicutt McGrath (2008) captures the essence of goal-setting philosophy when she states that ideally rehabilitation should be "patient centered *not* profession centered; participation/role based *not* impairment or activities based; interdisciplinary *not* multidisciplinary; goal directed *not* problem focused; individualized *not* programmatic" (p. 41; emphasis in original).

Awareness

"Awareness" is a term that can mean different things to different people. Broadly speaking, it is knowledge of a perception or a fact, but it can be interpreted in a number of ways.

Another term used regularly in neuropsychology is "anosognosia." The term was originally coined by Babinski (1914) to describe people who denied their hemiplegia, but is now more generally used to mean denial or lack of awareness of illness (Wilson, 2012). It can be differentiated from "anosodiaphoria," in which clients do not deny their illness but are unconcerned by their problems. The latter is associated with right-hemisphere lesions (Wilson, 2012). Also associated with right-hemisphere damage is "unilateral neglect" (a failure to report, respond to, or attend to stimuli on one side of space, usually the left; Heilman, Watson, Valenstein, & Goldberg, 1987).

When we talk about awareness after brain injury, however, we are usually referring to a person's knowledge and appreciation of his or her problems. It can be argued that rehabilitation is hampered when clients are unaware of their difficulties. This may be true in part, but lack of awareness does not preclude improvement in rehabilitation. After all, we can teach simple tasks to people in coma (Shiel, Wilson, Horn, Watson, & McLellan, 1993), and children with severe developmental learning difficulties can learn skills (Cullen, 1976); yet neither of these groups have good awareness. Nevertheless, those who have reasonable awareness of their difficulties are indeed more likely to benefit from rehabilitation. Ownsworth, McFarland, and McYoung (2000) describe a number of studies showing that individuals who have a good outcome after ABI are typically those who recognize and appreciate their limitations, set realistic goals, and actively participate in rehabilitation (Bergquist & Jackets, 1993; Deaton, 1986; Lam, McMahon, Priddy, & Gehred-Schultz, 1988; Prigatano, 1986). One of the main purposes of a holistic program—and this book—is to help people with brain injury become more aware of, and develop a better understanding of, the changes that have occurred as a result of the damage they have sustained (Trexler, Eberle, & Zappalá, 2000).

The starting point for rehabilitation is always to establish a client's level of awareness. The Crosson et al. (1989) pyramid model conceptualizes awareness by proposing three hierarchical levels: "intellectual," "emergent," and "anticipatory" awareness. Intellectual awareness involves recognition of deficits and an intellectual understanding of the implications of these deficits in everyday life; most clients will have some intellectual awareness of their difficulties on entering rehabilitation. Emergent awareness refers to an "in-the-moment" awareness, whereby individuals can recognize their difficulties as they occur. Finally, anticipatory awareness—regarded as the highest level of awareness—refers to an individual's ability to anticipate when difficulties may be experienced in the future (Barco, Crosson, Bolesta, Werts, & Stout, 1991). Once a client's initial level of awareness has been identified, interventions are targeted at moving up through these levels if possible.

In our experience, formal assessment has some contribution to building awareness. If the assessment is explained throughout and the client is aware of what each assessment is investigating, then the results can certainly contribute to developing intellectual awareness. Some assessments with good ecological validity (e.g., the Functional Assessment of Verbal Reasoning and Executive Skills; MacDonald, 1998) can imitate real-life tasks and allow someone to relate any struggles in the assessment to real-life experiences.

Questionnaires that explore a client's perceptions of difficulties can also offer valuable insights. The effect is cumulative if a measure is replicated with the client's significant other. For example, the La Trobe Communication Questionnaire (Douglas, O'Flaherty, & Snow,

2000) assesses both the client's and significant other's perceptions of the client's communication skills; the Patient Competency Rating Scale (Prigatano, 1986) asks clients to rate (on a scale of 1–5) how good they are at preparing their own meals, dressing themselves, keeping appointments, and so forth. An independent rater also completes the scale for each client, and this rating is used to determine whether the client has good or poor awareness of problems. Provided that the client's sense of safety is maintained, the feedback from the co-respondent can offer valuable insights. Video feedback can also be immensely valuable (see Keohane & Prince, Chapter 6, this volume).

Case Complexity

The content of any rehabilitation program provided is going to depend on a number of issues. These include the nature and severity of the brain damage sustained, the age of the person when seen, the person's age at the time of insult, and the status of the undamaged areas of the brain, as well as the person's premorbid cognitive functioning, personality, previous occupation, previous rehabilitation received, motivation, and family support. No client, however, is untreatable. Even those in a vegetative or minimally conscious state can benefit from rehabilitation (Wilson, Dhamapurkar, & Rose, 2016). Such clients cannot negotiate the goals, of course, but family members and other care providers working in the clients' best interests can consult as to the best way forward.

Robertson and Murre (1999) believe that the severity of brain damage determines whether or not rehabilitation is warranted. They suggest that those with mild lesions will recover spontaneously, that those with moderate lesions benefit from a retraining approach, and that those with severe lesions will require a compensatory approach. Although there may be some elements of truth in this belief, our opinion is that it is too simplistic and superficial. For example, the location of the lesion almost certainly plays a role in rehabilitation. Thus people with mild lesions in the frontal lobes may be more disadvantaged than people with severe lesions in the left anterior temporal lobe. The former group may have attention, planning, and organization problems precluding them from gaining the maximum benefit from the rehabilitation on offer, whereas the latter group, with language problems, may show considerable plasticity by transferring some of the language functions to the right hemisphere.

In addition, some people with a mild brain injury (defined as a confused state or loss of consciousness of less than 30 minutes, an initial Glasgow Coma Scale score of 13–15, and posttraumatic amnesia lasting less than 24 hours) can experience long-lasting problems. Ponsford et al. (2002) say that survivors of mild TBI can experience headache, dizziness, insomnia, reduced speed of thinking, concentration and memory problems, fatigue, irritability, anxiety, and depression, just like those with moderate or severe TBI. Furthermore, Ponsford et al. suggest that some symptoms may persist for years because of the stress of coping with reduced information-processing capacity.

As well as the nature and extent of the brain damage, we need to consider the influence of other factors on whether a person does well after a brain injury. Strong motivation, good family support systems, and the quality of rehabilitation available are likely to enhance success, whereas premorbid health problems, lack of social relationships, and reluctance to use strategies in the belief that this is somehow "cheating" or will prevent natural recovery may lead to limited improvement.

Group or Individual Work?

The importance of working with individuals is inherent in the rehabilitation program at OZC. We need to address each client's personal problems, involve him or her in the negotiation of goals, and find the best learning strategies for that individual. Nevertheless, all holistic treatment programs, including the one offered at OZC, provide both group and individual therapy (Trexler et al., 2000). We are all members of groups, be they family, work colleagues, social, political, religious, or leisure groups. Groups provide us with shared identities, roles, and peer support. We know that after brain injury many people experience a loss of roles and purpose, and experience a sense of isolation (Malley, Bateman, & Gracey, 2009); groups can help overcome this isolation. Many of the chapters in this book not only discuss individual work, but also suggest group work where this is possible.

Haslam et al. (2008) looked at individuals' memberships in multiple groups prior to stroke and found that continuity of social identity (maintenance of group membership after stroke) predicted well-being. In the authors' words, "Life satisfaction was associated both with multiple group memberships prior to stroke, and with maintenance of those group memberships" (p. 671).

In addition, therapists are invariably short of time, and one way of dealing with this is to treat people in groups rather than individually. It is also cheaper to treat several people at a time. A more important reason is that survivors of brain injury may benefit from interaction with others having similar problems. Sometimes they fear they are losing their sanity, and this fear may be alleviated by observing others with similar problems. Groups can reduce anxiety and distress. They can instill hope and show clients that they are not alone. It is often easier to accept advice from peers than from therapists, or to use strategies that peers are using rather than strategies recommended by the professional staff, so groups may lead to better learning of appropriate behavior. They may even result in altruism, such as supporting less able people within the group.

Group members may form friendships and reduce the feelings of social isolation. There is a saying that "nothing succeeds like success," so staff members running groups can ensure success within them by making the tasks appropriate to each member's ability level. This can further enhance members' self-esteem.

Groups also have face validity. That is, clients and families can see the point of groups and *believe* they are a good thing; this belief, in turn, can improve motivation to participate. Finally, groups are educative for the therapists running them. Considerable information can be gained by noting each client's responses to different strategies and observing which tasks are enjoyed or not enjoyed. Particular problems that arise can be observed and dealt with accordingly. In short, groups are a valuable treatment resource; they are important for people in distressing or demanding circumstances; and group acceptance and mutual support may bring about important clinical changes (Wilson, 2009).

We recognize that it is not always possible to run groups. This is especially likely to be true if therapists are working alone in the community. It may be possible to link with other local services to form support groups; alternatively, clients and caregivers can be encouraged to use online forums to share experiences.

CONCLUSIONS

By way of introduction to this workbook, this chapter has outlined the philosophy and core components of the OZC holistic rehabilitation program, on which the book is based. The chapter has described the principles of rehabilitation and stressed that the program's main purposes are to improve clients' functioning in everyday life and to help them reconstruct their identities. It has also looked at the principles of assessment and acknowledged the need to employ both standardized tests and behavioral or functional measures when therapists are evaluating a person's strengths and weaknesses. The chapter has acknowledged the importance of goal setting to plan rehabilitation and the value of making the goals meaningful and relevant to each client. Consideration has been given as well to the concept of awareness, which can mean different things to different people, and to how different types of awareness (or lack of it) might affect the design of a rehabilitation program. The chapter has taken a brief look at case complexity and the factors that can influence response to rehabilitation. Finally, it has addressed the importance of providing group as well as individual therapy.

My colleagues and I hope that this book will provide resources to support the rehabilitation of survivors of brain injury, and will provide information and understanding to their families, caregivers, and employers—especially in cases where survivors and their helpers may not be able to access the services of a specialist team.

REFERENCES

Austin, J. T., & Vancouver, J. B. (1996). Goal constructs in psychology: Structure, process, and content. *Psychological Bulletin, 120*(3), 338–375.

Babinski, J. (1914). Contribution to the study of mental disorders in organic cerebral hemiplegia (anosognosia). *Revue Neurologique (Paris), 27*, 845–848.

Barco, P. P., Crosson, B., Bolesta, M. M., Werts, D., & Stout, R. (1991). Training awareness and compensation in post-acute head injury rehabilitation. In J. S. Kreutzer & P. H. Wehman (Eds.), *Cognitive rehabilitation for persons with traumatic brain injury* (pp. 129–146). Baltimore: Brookes.

Ben-Yishay, Y. (1978). *Working approaches to the remediation of cognitive deficits in brain damaged persons* (Rehabilitation Monograph No. 59). New York: New York Medical Center.

Ben-Yishay, Y. (1996). Reflections on the evolution of the therapeutic milieu concept. *Neuropsychological Rehabilitation, 6*(4), 327–343.

Ben-Yishay, Y., & Prigatano, G. P. (1990). Cognitive remediation. In M. Rosenthal, E. R. Griffith, M. R. Bond, & J. D. Miller (Eds.), *Rehabilitation of the adult and child with traumatic brain injury* (2nd ed., pp. 393–409). Philadelphia: Davis.

Bergquist, T. F., & Jackets, M. P. (1993). Awareness and goal setting with the traumatically brain injured. *Brain Injury, 7*(3), 275–282.

Butler, G. (1998). Clinical formulation. *Comprehensive Clinical Psychology, 6*, 1–24.

Cicerone, K. D., Dahlberg, C., Malec, J. F., Langenbahn, D. M., Felicetti, T., Kneipp, S., . . .

Catanese, J. (2005). Evidence-based cognitive rehabilitation: Updated review of the literature from 1998 through 2002. *Archives of Physical Medicine and Rehabilitation, 86,* 1681–1692.

Cicerone, K. D., Langenbahn, D. M., Braden, C., Malec, J. F., Berquist, T., Azulay, J., . . . Ashman, T. (2011). Evidence-based cognitive rehabilitation: Updated review of the literature from 2003 through 2008. *Archives of Physical Medicine and Rehabilitation, 92,* 519–530.

Cicerone, K. D., Mott, T., Azulay, J., Sharlow-Galella, M. A., Elmo, W. J., Paradise, S., et al. (2008). A randomized controlled trial of holistic neuropsychologic rehabilitation after traumatic brain injury. *Archives of Physical Medicine and Rehabilitation, 89*(12), 2239–2249.

Collicutt McGrath, J. (2008). Post-acute in-patient rehabilitation. In A. Tyerman & N. S. King (Eds.), *Psychological approaches to rehabilitation after traumatic brain injury* (pp. 39–64). Malden, MA: Wiley-Blackwell.

Cope, D. N., Cole, J. R., Hali, K. M., & Barkan, H. (1991). Brain injury: Analysis of outcome in a post-acute rehabilitation system: Part 2. Subanalyses. *Brain Injury, 5*(2), 127–139.

Crosson, B., Barco, P. P., Vallejo, C. A., Bolesta, M. M., Cooper, P. V., Werts, D., & Brobeck, T. C. (1989). Awareness of compensation in post-acute head injury rehabilitation. *Journal of Head Trauma Rehabilitation, 4,* 46–54.

Cullen, K. J. (1976). A six-year controlled trial of prevention of children's behavior disorders. *Journal of Pediatrics, 88*(4), 662–666.

Deaton, A. V. (1986). Denial in the aftermath of traumatic head injury: Its manifestations, measurement, and treatment. *Rehabilitation Psychology, 31*(4), 231–240.

Diller, L. L. (1976). A model for cognitive retraining in rehabilitation. *The Clinical Psychologist, 29,* 13–15.

Douglas, J., O'Flaherty, C. A., & Snow, P. C. (2000). Measuring perception of communicative ability: The development and evaluation of the La Trobe Communication Questionnaire. *Aphasiology, 14*(3), 251–268.

Evans, J. J. (2012). Goal setting during rehabilitation early and late after acquired brain injury. *Current Opinion in Neurology, 25*(6), 651–655.

Friel, J. C. (2008). A randomized controlled trial of holistic neuropsychologic rehabilitation after traumatic brain injury. *Archives of Physical Medicine Rehabilitation, 89,* 2239–2249.

Gracey, F., Evans, J. J., & Malley, D. (2009). Capturing process and outcome in complex rehabilitation interventions: A "Y-shaped" model. *Neuropsychological Rehabilitation, 19*(6), 867–890.

Haslam, C., Holme, A., Haslam, S. A., Iyer, A., Jetten, J., & Williams, W. H. (2008). Maintaining group memberships: Social identity continuity predicts well-being after stroke. *Neuropsychological Rehabilitation, 18*(5–6), 671–691.

Haughey, D. (2011, May 4). Setting smarter goals in 7 easy steps. Retrieved from *www.projectsmart. co.uk.*

Heilman, K. M., Watson, R. T., Valenstein, E., & Goldberg, M. E. (1987). Attention: Behavior and neural mechanisms. In F. Plum (Ed.), *Handbook of physiology: Section 1. The nervous system. Vol. 5. Higher functions of the brain* (pp. 461–481). Bethesda, MD: American Physiological Society.

Houts, P. S., & Scott, R. A. (1975). *Goal planning with developmentally disabled persons: Procedures for developing an individualized client plan.* University Park: Pennsylvania State University, Hershey Department of Behavioral Science. (ERIC Document Reproduction Service No. ED 119431)

Kersten, P., McPherson, K. M., Kayes, N. M., Theadom, A., & McCambridge, A. (2015). Bridging the goal intention–action gap in rehabilitation: A study of if–then implementation intentions in neurorehabilitation. *Disability and Rehabilitation, 37*(12), 1073–1081.

Lam, C. S., McMahon, B. T., Priddy, D. A., & Gehred-Schultz, A. (1988). Deficit awareness and treatment performance among traumatic head injury adults. *Brain Injury, 2*(3), 235–242.

Levack, W. M., Weatherall, M., Hay-Smith, E. J. C., Dean, S. G., McPherson, K., & Siegert, R. J.

(2015). Goal setting and strategies to enhance goal pursuit for adults with acquired disability participating in rehabilitation. *Cochrane Database of Systematic Reviews, 20*(7), CD009727.

MacDonald, S. (1998). *Functional assessment of verbal reasoning and executive strategies.* Guelph, Canada: Clinical Publishing.

Malley, D., Bateman, A., & Gracey, F. (2009). Practically based project groups. In B. A. Wilson, F. Gracey, J. J. Evans, & A. Bateman, *Neuropsychological rehabilitation: Theory, models, therapy and outcome* (pp. 164–180). Cambridge, UK: Cambridge University Press.

McLellan, D. L. (1991). Functional recovery and the principles of disability medicine. *Clinical Neurology, 1,* 768–790.

McMillan, T. M., & Sparkes, C. (1999). Goal planning and neurorehabilitation: The Wolfson Neurorehabilitation Centre approach. *Neuropsychological Rehabilitation, 9*(3–4), 241–251.

Mehlbye, J., & Larsen, A. (1994). Social and economic consequences of brain damage in Denmark. In A.-L. Christensen & B. P. Uzzell (Eds.), *Brain injury and neuropsychological rehabilitation: International perspectives* (pp. 257–267). Hillsdale, NJ: Erlbaum.

Nair, K. S., & Wade, D. T. (2003). Satisfaction of members of interdisciplinary rehabilitation teams with goal planning meetings. *Archives of Physical Medicine and Rehabilitation, 84*(11), 1710–1713.

Ownsworth, T. L., McFarland, K., & McYoung, R. (2000). Self-awareness and psychosocial functioning following acquired brain injury: An evaluation of a group support programme. *Neuropsychological Rehabilitation, 10*(5), 465–484.

Ponsford, J., Willmott, C., Rothwell, A., Cameron, P., Kelly, A. M., Nelms, R., & Curran, C. (2002). Impact of early intervention on outcome following mild head injury in adults. *Journal of Neurology, Neurosurgery and Psychiatry, 73*(3), 330–332.

Prigatano, G. P. (1986). Personality and psychosocial consequences of brain injury. In G. P. Prigatano, D. J. Fordyce, H. K. Zeiner, J. R. Roueche, M. Pepping, & B. C. Wood (Eds.), *Neuropsychological rehabilitation after brain injury* (pp. 29–50). Baltimore: Johns Hopkins University Press.

Prigatano, G. P. (1999). *Principles of neuropsychological rehabilitation.* New York: Oxford University Press.

Robertson, I. H., & Murre, J. M. (1999). Rehabilitation of brain damage: Brain plasticity and principles of guided recovery. *Psychological Bulletin, 125*(5), 544–575.

Sherratt, S., Worrall, L., Hersh, D., Howe, T., & Davidson, B. (2015). Goals and goal setting for people with aphasia, their family members and clinicians. In R. J. Siegert & W. M. M. Levack (Eds.), *Rehabilitation goal setting: Theory, practice and evidence* (pp. 325–343). Boca Raton, FL: CRC Press.

Shiel, A., Wilson, B. A., Horn, S., Watson, M., & McLellan, L. (1993). *The Wessex Head Injury Matrix (WHIM).* Bury St. Edmunds, UK: Thames Valley Test Company.

Sundberg, N. D., & Tyler, L. E. (1962). *Clinical psychology: An introduction to research and practice.* New York: Appleton-Century-Crofts.

Trexler, L. E., Eberle, R., & Zappalá, G. (2000). Models and programs of the Center for Neuropsychological Rehabilitation. In A.-L. Christensen & B. P. Uzzell (Eds.), *International handbook of neuropsychological rehabilitation* (pp. 215–229). New York: Kluwer Academic/Plenum.

Wilson, B. A. (1997). Cognitive rehabilitation: How it is and how it might be. *Journal of the International Neuropsychological Society, 3*(5), 487–496.

Wilson, B. A. (2009). Kate: Cognitive recovery and emotional adjustment in a young woman who was unresponsive for several months. In B. A. Wilson, F. Gracey, J. J. Evans, & A. Bateman, *Neuropsychological rehabilitation: Theory, models, therapy and outcomes.* Cambridge, UK: Cambridge University Press.

Wilson, B. A. (2012). Book review. In C. A. Noggle, R. S. Dean, & A. M. Horton Jr. (Eds.), The encyclopedia of neuropsychological disorders. *Neuropsychological Rehabilitation, 22*(4), 650–651.

Wilson, B. A., Dhamapurkar, S., & Rose, A., (2016). *Surviving brain injury after assault: Gary's story.* Hove, UK: Psychology Press.

Wilson, B. A., & Evans, J. J. (2002). Does cognitive rehabilitation work?: Clinical and economic considerations and outcomes. In G. Prigatano & N. H. Pliskin (Eds.), *Clinical neuropsychology and cost–outcome research: An introduction* (pp. 329–349). Hove, UK: Psychology Press.

Wilson, B. A., Gracey, F., Evans, J. J., & Bateman, A. (2009). *Neuropsychological rehabilitation: Theory, models, therapy and outcomes.* Cambridge, UK: Cambridge University Press.

Wilson, B. A., Robertson, C., & Mole, J. (2015). *Identity unknown: How acute brain disease can destroy knowledge of oneself and others.* Hove, UK: Psychology Press.

Yemm, G. (2013). *The Financial Times essential guide to leading your team: How to set goals, measure performance and reward talent.* Harlow, UK: Pearson Education.

Ylvisaker, M., & Feeney, T. (2000). Reconstruction of identity after brain injury. *Brain Impairment, 1*(1), 12–28.

Formulation Template

Key Relationships	Brain Pathology	Social/Medical Factors	Cognition

Communication	Mood	Sensory/Perceptual Factors	Physical Factors

Insight	Functional Consequences	Losses

From *The Brain Injury Rehabilitation Workbook*, edited by Rachel Winson, Barbara A. Wilson, and Andrew Bateman. Copyright © 2017 The Guilford Press. Permission to photocopy this handout is granted to purchasers of this book for personal use or for use with individual clients (see copyright page for details). Purchasers can download additional copies of this handout (see the box at the end of the table of contents).

CHAPTER 2

Introduction to Brain Anatomy and Mechanisms of Injury

Emily Grader
Andrew Bateman

A lack of understanding of brain injury among survivors is an issue that can impede engagement in rehabilitation. Information about an individual's brain injury may be embedded in technical language. Clients may have frequently met with professionals or read their own reports, but understood very little. Their limited understanding, along with the stigma attached to being "brain-damaged" or having cognitive impairments, can be a barrier to successful rehabilitation. This potential barrier can be overcome by helping clients to understand—albeit at a very basic level—how the brain works, how their particular types of injury have affected their brain function, and how this can account for difficulties they may be experiencing day to day. This understanding can then be shared appropriately with friends and families.

Educating clients about brain injury requires gathering both general background information to provide a context, and specific personalized information from the clients' medical records (which can be requested from the clients' general practitioners or primary care providers). The medical records are likely to have been written in technical language; one of a clinician's key tasks may be to help simplify the records into concepts accessible to the clients.

This chapter provides basic-level information about brain anatomy and some mechanisms of injury, both in simple written form and through figures (with labels for clinicians) and handouts (with simplified labels, to be maximally accessible to clients). Suggestions are also given for how to support clients in finding out more about their particular types of injury, both from their specialist clinicians and from other sources of information.

CLINICAL RISK ASSESSMENT

It is advisable for clinicians to consider the risks associated with this work. In particular, some clients may be seeking to justify problems as "due to my brain injury," whereas the changes in their behavior and experience may have their roots elsewhere—for example, in depression, anxiety, or reactions to their recent experiences. Furthermore, it is important to consider the timing of any intervention aimed at increasing clients' understanding of brain injury. The right moment for each client is found through dialogue and goal setting. If an intervention is provided too early, the information can be overwhelming, which may erode a client's hope and optimism and undermine other rehabilitation efforts. Clients have reported experiencing dips in mood as their understanding and awareness of their difficulties increase; therapists should be prepared to offer extra psychological support or to refer clients to appropriate services if such dips should occur.

At the same time, it is important for therapists and clients alike to be aware that sometimes not everything can be explained simply. For example, predicting and identifying specific emotional reactions from specific lesion locations can be very difficult, mainly because individual brain regions contribute to multiple emotions and may be involved in more than one functional circuit. For example, research studies have demonstrated that the amygdala is associated with both positive and negative emotions, as well as with basic emotions such as fear and disgust (Baas, Alemana, & Kahn, 2004). Findings like these, which fail to demonstrate one-to-one correspondences between discrete emotions or affective dimensions and specific brain areas, seem to indicate that complex networks (i.e., patterns of connections between brain structures) could potentially provide a more appropriate level of explanation—something that is not always easy to explain.

GROUP WORK

If circumstances permit, it can be beneficial to cover the information provided in this chapter in a small study group. A group of brain injury survivors can share information about their injuries and experiences, and discuss their interpretations of the information provided. We suggest a round-table seminar format in which the information is presented via PowerPoint slides, and the clients are provided with copies of the slides and encouraged to make notes. Discussion and questions are encouraged at all times, particularly when what is being presented relates to the clients' own experience. The pace and structure of the group will also depend on the clients' needs and group dynamics.

A possible syllabus for the group might follow four key themes:

1. Anatomy
2. Mechanisms of injury
3. Stages of recovery
4. Common consequences of injury

The first three themes are covered in this chapter; consequences of injury (from a cognitive and emotional viewpoint) are covered in other chapters. It can be helpful to ask clients to complete the questionnaire in Handout 2.1* before the group sessions begin, to gauge their current level of knowledge/confidence and any areas of particular interest. The questionnaire can be repeated once the syllabus is completed, as a crude way of measuring change.

ANATOMY

The aim of providing basic neuroanatomical information is to introduce clients to the structures of the brain and associated terminology. Clients and their families may have heard various terms used in the course of the clients' care, and often find it helpful to learn more about the regions mentioned. With this understanding, many clients report that they are able to begin making sense of what has happened to them.

Clearly neuroanatomy is a very big topic, with many specialists dedicating years of study to a particular region. The challenge of providing enough detail to be interesting has to be balanced with keeping things simple enough to be understandable. In this chapter, the focus is on providing information at a basic level. Clients with strong background knowledge can be helped to find appropriate textbooks and other resources in order to achieve a more in-depth scientific understanding. A list of some useful resources is provided at the end of the chapter.

Brain Cells

The brain is made up of billions of tiny cells known as neurons. Under a microscope, a neuron appears to have three sections:

1. *Dendrites and cell body.* The cell body controls the activity of the cell. The dendrites, or dendrons, are branches that transmit messages to the cell body from other cells.
2. *Axon and myelin sheath.* Nerve impulses travel along the axon, which is coated in a fatty substance called myelin, which increases the speed at which impulses travel.
3. *Axon terminals.* These are the junctions between the neuron and other neurons, across which neurotransmitters pass.

An illustration is provided in Figure 2.1, and a version of this illustration with simplified labels for clients' use is provided in Handout 2.2. The term "gray matter" is commonly used in talking about the brain. What this refers to is regions of the brain comprising predominantly cell bodies (gray matter), as opposed to areas consisting predominantly of axons (white matter). The white matter appears white because the myelin sheath surrounding the axons contains a fat that looks white, and the cell bodies can look gray by comparison.

---

*All handouts are at the end of the chapter.

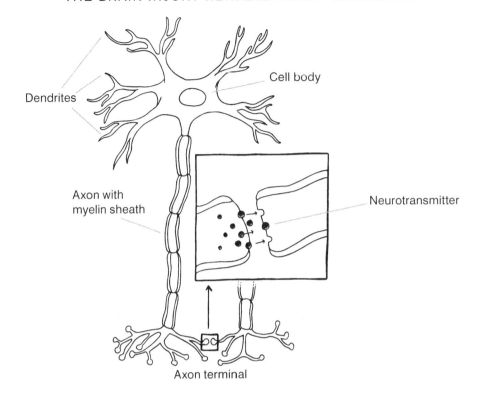

Dendrites

Cell body

Axon with
myelin sheath

Neurotransmitter

Axon terminal

FIGURE 2.1. Neurons.

Neurons communicate with each other by releasing chemical messengers (called neurotransmitters), such as dopamine. As the brain develops, it forms specialized communication pathways or networks, which allow information to be processed and interpreted. In recent years, as the term "neuroplasticity" has entered public consciousness, many survivors ask about its relevance to their rehabilitation. It is important to understand that neuronal connections are continually changing throughout our lives. Connections strengthen or weaken according to demands and stimulation. After injury, rehabilitation is one type of demand that can help shape how the brain is recovering. An engaging article on this topic was recently published on the Wellcome Trust's Mosaic website (Storr, 2015).

Skull, Meninges, and Cerebrospinal Fluid

The brain is protected from the external environment by the skull, three membranes (meninges) and the cerebrospinal fluid (CSF). The skull is made of bone, and although it appears smooth from the outside, the inside contains many ridges—which can have an abrasive effect, particularly during a traumatic brain injury (see "Mechanisms of Injury," on page 22). Between two of the meninges (the arachnoid and pia mater) is the subarachnoid space, containing a rich blood supply to the brain, and CSF. This space helps to protect the brain by acting as a shock absorber, as well as circulating nutrients and removing waste products from the brain (see Figure 2.2 and Handout 2.3).

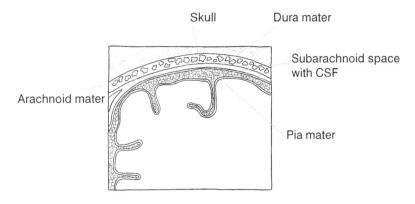

FIGURE 2.2. Protection for the brain.

Brain Stem

At the base of the brain is the brain stem. This connects the brain with the spinal cord and the rest of the body. It is also the area of the brain responsible for the majority of autonomic or unconscious functions, such as breathing, swallowing, cardiac function, temperature regulation, and sleep–wakefulness.

Cerebral Hemispheres

The bulk of the brain is a wrinkled structure known as the cerebrum. The cerebrum is made up of two cerebral hemispheres (right and left), which communicate via a structure known as the corpus callosum. Each cerebral hemisphere can be said to be (mainly) responsible for one half of the body. Interestingly, the left hemisphere is responsible for the right side, and the right hemisphere for the left.

Each hemisphere consists of four lobes (see Figure 2.3 and Handout 2.4). Damage to any of the parts of the brain can affect a person's overall capacity to function effectively, in addition to specific problems linked to the regions described here.

Frontal Lobe

As its name suggests, the frontal lobe is the lobe at the front of the brain, located beneath the forehead. It is generally considered as the area most responsible for executive functions (i.e., planning, organizing, self-monitoring, initiating, and adapting; see Winegardner, Chapter 5, this volume). It has also been associated with personality, and many people report personality changes after damage to this area. Furthermore, at the very back of the frontal lobe is the motor cortex, which controls movement of muscle groups.

Temporal Lobe

The temporal lobe in each hemisphere is located behind the ear on that side. It is generally considered as the area of the brain where long-term memory, auditory processing, and understanding language occur.

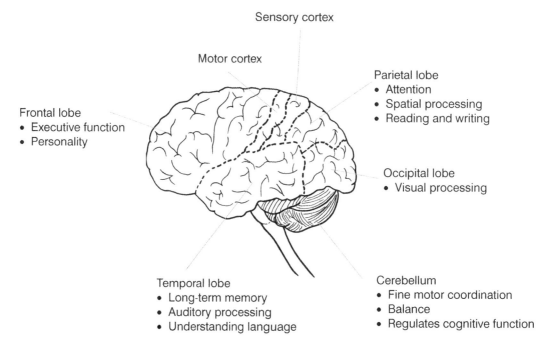

Sensory cortex

Motor cortex

Parietal lobe
- Attention
- Spatial processing
- Reading and writing

Frontal lobe
- Executive function
- Personality

Occipital lobe
- Visual processing

Temporal lobe
- Long-term memory
- Auditory processing
- Understanding language

Cerebellum
- Fine motor coordination
- Balance
- Regulates cognitive function

FIGURE 2.3. Brain regions.

Parietal Lobe

The parietal lobe in each hemisphere is located at the back of the brain, above the ear on that side. It is generally considered as the area of the brain responsible for attention, spatial processing and perception, reading, and writing. At the very front of the parietal lobe is a region known as the sensory cortex, which receives messages from sensory receptors around the body.

Occipital Lobe

The occipital lobe is located at the very back of the brain. It is responsible for basic visual processing.

Cerebellum

The cerebellum is the region tucked under the cerebral hemispheres at the base of the brain. It is responsible for fine motor coordination and balance. A less well-known role is that it plays an important function in regulating the cognitive tasks of the cerebrum.

Limbic System

In the middle of the brain is a set of structures known collectively as the limbic system. This primitive system is often considered the "old brain," responsible for our basic perceptions of emotions and instinctive responses to them. More details are provided by Ford in Chapter 8 of this volume. Some important structures within the limbic system include the following:

- *Amygdala.* An almond-shaped structure linked to our automatic emotional responses, especially fear, aggression, and pleasure.
- *Hippocampus.* A structure critically involved in making memories.
- *Pituitary gland.* The master gland that secretes hormones to control growth and metabolism.
- *Hypothalamus.* A structure that acts rather like the body's thermostat, helping to monitor and maintain the right conditions for the body to function properly (including temperature, pulse, digestion, blood pressure, breathing, and heart rate).

It has also been shown that the frontal lobes have strong connections with the limbic system and are responsible for monitoring its instinctive responses and evaluating whether these are appropriate.

Blood Supply

The role of blood is to bring oxygen and nutrients to cells to enable them to function. Blood also removes waste products such as carbon dioxide from the cells, preventing toxicity. It is important that brain cells receive a steady supply of blood; they begin to die if they are deprived of an adequate supply of oxygen for even a few minutes. The circulation system in the skull is therefore crucially important, and the brain is supplied by a dense network of blood vessels (see Figure 2.4 and Handout 2.5). The main arteries supplying the brain join

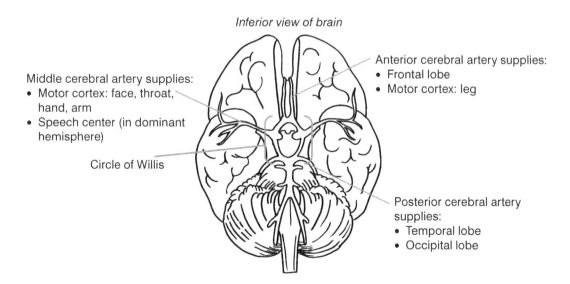

FIGURE 2.4. The brain's blood supply.

to form a ring at its base, from which smaller arteries arise and spread through the brain; thus, if one of the main arteries is blocked, blood can still continue to circulate.

MECHANISMS OF INJURY

An acquired brain injury (ABI) is an injury to the brain that has occurred at some time after birth. Here we discuss some of the most common causes of ABI.

Trauma

A traumatic brain injury (TBI) is an injury caused by direct trauma to the head. TBIs can largely be categorized into two groups:

1. *Closed.* The skull remains intact. Examples of closed head injuries include road traffic accidents and falls that do not penetrate the skull.
2. *Open.* The skull is penetrated and the brain is exposed to the external environment. An example of an open injury is a gunshot to the head.

The moment of injury is the starting point for a chain of events causing damage to the brain. A closed head injury is caused by hitting one's head against a hard object, such as a car windshield or a wall. The associated violent movement of the soft brain tissue as it bangs against the hard skull results in bruising, bleeding, and/or swelling of the tissues. This injury affects a wide area of the brain and causes damage to many nerve pathways. Road traffic accidents often result in what is known as diffuse axonal injury (DAI), due to the rapid acceleration and deceleration movements of the brain within the skull. This means that damage occurs due to tearing of nerve cells in quite widespread areas of the brain, which may not show up on brain scans. However, DAI can significantly interfere with the function of the brain even in mild cases, partly because it affects the ability of different parts of the brain to communicate with each other as effectively as before.

A TBI can also result in damage to a specific region of the brain (focal damage). For example, a blow to the left side of the head can cause damage to the left temporal lobe. In what is known as a coup–contrecoup injury, damage occurs at the site of the impact and also at the opposite side from the point of external trauma, as the brain ricochets from one internal surface of the skull to another.

Further/secondary injury to the brain can follow the initial trauma. Some types of such injury are described below.

Anoxia

The brain may be starved of oxygen as a result of blocked airways, excessive bleeding, or respiratory arrest at the time of the trauma. Neurons die quickly without oxygen. A lack of oxygen to the brain can have a widespread effect and is often referred to as diffuse anoxic damage. Focal anoxic damage may be found in particularly circulation-rich areas of the brain.

Inflammation

Swelling is a natural reaction to any injury and is an important part of the body's recovery. However, as the brain (especially in closed head injuries) is encapsulated by the skull, the pressure within the skull increases when the brain swells. This pressure increase squashes the brain and causes widespread damage to delicate neurons. Inflammation can also restrict the supply of oxygen to the brain by constricting blood vessels. In an intensive care setting, swelling inside the brain is monitored carefully, and a piece of the skull may need to be removed to relieve pressure (craniotomy).

Infection

Open TBIs are particularly vulnerable to infections, as the brain is directly exposed to the infectious organisms in the external environment. Infections can cause further direct damage to brain cells, as well as increasing the likelihood of swelling as the body's inflammatory response fights the infection.

Hemorrhage and Hematoma

If blood vessels are torn during the traumatic event, blood can leak into the space between the brain and the skull (this is called a traumatic subarachnoid hemorrhage). Sometimes a blood clot or hematoma can form. If the hematoma is large, it can increase the pressure on the brain, causing further damage.

Vascular Events

Stroke

A stroke occurs when the blood supply to a part of the brain is disrupted. This can result from either a blockage by a blood clot, fat globule, or air bubble (known as an ischemic stroke) or a bleed inside or on the surface of the brain (a hemorrhagic stroke). As the blood supply is disrupted, the neurons in that particular area do not receive the oxygen and nutrients they need to survive. The consequences of a stroke depend on the brain area(s) affected.

Aneurysm

An aneurysm is a weak point in the wall of a blood vessel. Under pressure, the weak point can stretch and balloon out, with the risk that it will burst.

Arteriovenous Malformation

Arteriovenous malformation (AVM) is a congenital tangle of blood vessels with abnormal connections between high-pressure arteries and low-pressure veins. The tangle makes the vessels prone to bleeding, which causes a stroke. Eighty percent of people with an AVM have no symptoms.

Other Causes of Injury

Infections

Infections can cause damage to the brain by directly affecting brain cells and via swelling. Increased pressure within the cranium can potentially mean that blood cannot successfully flow through the capillaries (fine blood vessels) supplying the brain. Meningitis is a bacterial or viral infection located in the membranes surrounding the brain. Encephalitis is an infection within the brain itself; it can be caused by a virus but is sometimes the result of an autoimmune reaction.

Tumors

Tumors are abnormal growths of cells within the brain. A malignant tumor is fast-growing and invasive, and can destroy surrounding healthy brain tissue. Although a benign tumor is slower-growing and not invasive, it can nevertheless compress or damage surrounding healthy tissue.

Hypoxia/Anoxia

The brain may also be damaged as a result of oxygen deprivation, either due to an acute event (such as cardiac/respiratory arrest) or over a period of time (e.g., chronic sleep apnea).

STAGES OF RECOVERY

Discussing the process of recovering from brain injury can be particularly important for clients who have experienced TBI, who may have little or no memory of the time they spent in intensive care during the acute phase. Developing an understanding of some of the behaviors commonly seen immediately after TBI can also help families reframe this experience, which may have been bewildering or distressing at the time.

Coma

Coma is a state of depressed consciousness, in which a person shows reduced responsiveness to stimuli. A coma may be medically induced after a severe injury to minimize the demands on the brain, allowing it to rest and recover. There are different levels of coma, meaning that individuals may be more or less responsive, and coma can last any length of time from hours to days to weeks. The duration and grade of the coma (according to the widely used Glasgow Coma Scale) can be used as a very rough estimate of the severity of the injury.

Contrary to the depictions often seen in films or on TV, in which a person is fully lucid upon first regaining consciousness, the process of emerging from coma is in fact gradual. Clients gradually become able to respond to certain stimuli and to follow commands. They may be confused, agitated, disoriented, or disinhibited to begin with.

Posttraumatic Amnesia

The next stage of recovery is posttraumatic amnesia (PTA), in which a person may be conscious and appear lucid, but has difficulty retaining information from moment to moment. Clients may be disoriented to time, place, or person, and can continue to be disinhibited or aggressive, which can be challenging for family members to witness. PTA is considered to have resolved once a person is able to answer a series of basic questions (e.g., the person's name, address, and date of birth; where he or she is; who the prime minister or president is).

Neurological Recovery

Brain cells do not regenerate in the same way as other tissues, such as skin and bone. However, the brain does have the capacity to grow new connections between cells (rather as new roads might be built in a city center that has been damaged in an earthquake). This is known as "neuroplasticity"; the younger a person with brain damage is, the more able the brain is to develop new neural pathways. Stimulation supports the creation of these pathways, which is why early rehabilitation after brain injury is so important. Most change is seen in the first 6 months after injury, though improvements can be noted 2 years afterward, with some clients continuing to improve as much as 5 years after injury (Fleminger & Ponsford, 2005). Nevertheless, as Fleminger and Ponsford suggest, it is important to bear in mind that adjustment after brain injury is a complex process, and to be aware that lasting neuropsychiatric difficulties are not uncommon.

CONSOLIDATING LEARNING

Suggestions are given below for activities to illustrate some of the points covered in this chapter, and to support more active learning styles. Be sure to take into account your clients' abilities before engaging in these, as not all tasks will be appropriate for everyone. You may also wish to use interactive brain models and online video clips to support learning (some sources for these are suggested at the end of this chapter).

- Get clients to play reaction time games (such games are readily available online) to illustrate the speed of nerve impulses.
- The multitude of neural connections can be demonstrated by giving each client a sheet of paper with a number of dots on it, and asking the clients to join every dot to every other one on the sheet.
- The role of CSF can be illustrated by shaking an egg first inside an empty plastic container and then inside another filled with water. The container represents the skull, the egg represents the brain, and the water serves the same function as CSF. The eggshell usually cracks when the container is shaken without water, but remains intact when water is added.
- Some clients may enjoy sculpting a brain from modeling clay, using a different color for each region.

- Visual perception can be explored by using a range of optical illusions (again, these are freely available on the Internet).

- Auditory perception can be investigated by playing a range of sound effects and asking clients to identify them.

- Cerebellar control of balance can be explained by asking clients to stand on a "wobble board" while you talk them through the process.

- Sensory cortex function can be explored by using a bag containing objects of varying sizes and textures (e.g., a paper clip, a cotton ball, a piece of sandpaper, a feather, a piece of leather or silk) and asking clients to guess what each object is by feeling it.

- Asking clients to write their names on a piece of paper while watching the pen in a mirror can be an interesting way of exploring spatial awareness and writing skills.

- We acknowledge that skills are not simply mapped to a single brain region; nevertheless, the following exercise can help people to remember and visualize their functional neuroanatomy and to understand how their injuries have led to their difficulties. Ask clients to think of people they know—they can be either personal acquaintances or celebrity figures—who personify particular skill sets relating to a given brain region. For example:

  o Athletes such as football or soccer players and golfers are very accurate at judging distance and depth, demonstrating strong spatial awareness and processing skills (parietal lobes).
  o Business leaders often have skills in organizing and strategic planning (frontal lobes).
  o Artists, writers, and musicians can have great emotional sensitivity (limbic system).

Some clients find it helpful to conceptualize these figures as "heroes" or "heroines" as they work toward improving their skills in a particular area. (For more suggestions, see Gracey, Prince, & Winson, Chapter 9, this volume.)

- When explaining executive functions, try presenting clients with a role-play scenario, illustrating various difficulties with executive functioning. For example, one staff member invites another over for a cup of coffee, then struggles to sequence the steps involved: he or she does not initiate putting the coffee on, makes coffee instead of tea after the visitor has changed his or her order to tea, has forgotten to buy milk, and is disinhibited in conversation. If the performance of the staff member simulating brain damage is sufficiently exaggerated, clients should be able to spot the difficulties.

PREPARING CLIENTS TO ASK THEIR DOCTORS QUESTIONS

In this chapter, we have outlined some basic information on neuroanatomy and brain injury that may be provided as part of a rehabilitation intervention. As mentioned above, individuals vary in the level of detail that they require, but most are curious about what brain scans and medical notes can tell them about their recovery.

We would encourage therapists to help clients become as expert as possible in their own conditions, by "translating" medical information into ordinary language and by making links between the anatomy of clients' particular injuries and their day-to-day experiences. This may involve gathering information from a range of services involved in a client's care. It is important to note that medical patients in the United Kingdom have the right to access their clinical records, although it may be necessary to write a formal letter to request access to the information. The website of the Information Commissioner's Office provides an example template for this (*https://ico.org.uk/for-the-public/health*). In the United States, patients have the right to inspect any of their medical records that are held by health plans and health care providers covered by the Health Insurance Portability and Accountability Act (HIPAA) Privacy Rule. Even if patients have not paid for the services they have received, providers cannot deny them access to their records. Charges can be made for reasonable expenses incurred in copying and delivering the records, although a provider cannot charge a fee for searching for or retrieving records. More information is available on a page of the U.S. Department of Health and Human Services website (*www.hhs.gov/ocr/privacy/hipaa/understanding/consumers/medicalrecords.html*).

It may also be necessary to refer clients to a wider multidisciplinary team of specialists (neuroradiologists, neuroendocrinologists, neuro-ophthalmologists, or neurosurgeons) for answers to questions that are beyond the scope of the rehabilitation team. By becoming empowered and asking carefully planned questions, clients can reduce their sense of uncertainty about their conditions. Some frequently asked questions are listed below; the answers to these questions are highly individualized, which is why it is appropriate to seek advice from an appropriate clinician who has a good overview of a particular client's condition.

"How much damage has my brain sustained?"

"I've been told that after a given period [e.g., 6 weeks, 6 months, 2 years], my brain will stop recovering. Is this true?"

"Will I have another stroke?"

"Will I develop dementia?"

"When will I be back to normal?"

"How can I train my brain?"

"Are there dietary changes I can make to improve my brain?"

"What medication should I be taking to improve my brain?"

"Why am I on this [particular named] medication/dose?"

BRINGING IT ALL TOGETHER

In this chapter, we have outlined some information on anatomy and the mechanics of brain injury to help clients begin to make sense of their experiences. It can be helpful for each client to create a portfolio, beginning with a document that contains personalized information about his or her own condition, linking information about brain structure and pathology to functional difficulties that the client is experiencing (see Handout 2.6). This document, and the portfolio as a whole, can be added to as the client learns more. Each chapter of this workbook provides handouts that can contribute to clients' understanding of the challenges they face, as well as their strengths. The portfolio can be shared with family members or friends as each client chooses.

Alternatively, clients can undertake various creative projects as a way of developing their understanding of what has happened to them. For example, they may wish to do one of the following:

- Create a timeline, either as an artwork or mixed media piece, using metaphor as appropriate (e.g., a train journey through mountains and valleys to represent high and low points in their recovery).
- Make a collage of photographs of important life events.
- Produce a film telling their stories, or describing a day in their lives after brain injury.
- Create a model relating to an aspect of the brain (e.g., a wooden brain jigsaw puzzle showing the lobes).
- Write a song/compose a piece of music.

REFERENCES

Baas, D., Alemana, A., & Kahn, R. S. (2004). Lateralization of amygdala activation: A systematic review of functional neuroimaging studies. *Brain Research Reviews, 45*, 96–103.

Fleminger, S., & Ponsford, J. (2005). Long-term outcome after traumatic brain injury. *British Medical Journal, 331*(7530), 1419–1420.

Storr, W. (2015, November 17). Can you think yourself into a different person? Retrieved from *http://mosaicscience.com/story/neuroplasticity*

USEFUL RESOURCES

3D Brain App is a useful interactive resource for the iPhone; it allows the user to explore brain anatomy and function (*https://itunes.apple.com/gb/app/3d-brain/id331399332?mt=8*).

The Harvard Brain Atlas (*www.med.harvard.edu/aanlib*) offers detailed scans of healthy, normally aging, and injured brains.

The Atlas of the Brain in Stereotaxic Space (*www.thehumanbrain.info/brain*) is an interactive resource that allows the user to browse sections of the brain in all planes in both photographic and diagrammatic form.

Coloring books with drawings of the brain are useful resources for both clinicians and clients. With the recent increase in the popularity of coloring books generally, several such books are now available. One example is *The Human Brain Coloring Book* by Diamond, Scheibel, and Elson.

Excellent, high-quality anatomical models of the brain can be sourced from the British firm Adam, Rouilly (*www.adam-rouilly.co.uk/products.aspx?cid=201*). In the United States, such models are commercially available from AnatomyNow (*www.anatomynow.com*) or from Shop Anatomical (*www.anatomy-models.shopanatomical.com*).

Understanding Brain Injury: Group Questionnaire

Please write down here some things you would like to find out about (e.g., terms you have heard during your medical care or rehabilitation to date).

_____

_____

_____

_____

Now please use the scales below to rate your current satisfaction with the knowledge you have, as well as other aspects of your knowledge. On each scale, give a rating from 1 to 10, using the labels to guide you.

I am satisfied with my current level of knowledge about my brain injury and its consequences.

1	2	3	4	5	6	7	8	9	10

Not at all satisfied   Completely satisfied

Comments: _____

I have a basic understanding of how the brain works and affects my day-to-day abilities.

1	2	3	4	5	6	7	8	9	10

No understanding   Excellent understanding

Comments: _____

I know where to find out more information about my brain injury and its consequences.

1	2	3	4	5	6	7	8	9	10

No idea   Very clear idea

Comments: _____

I have unanswered questions about my brain injury.

1	2	3	4	5	6	7	8	9	10

Many questions   No questions

Comments: _____

I feel confident in my ability to explain my brain injury and its consequences to others.

1	2	3	4	5	6	7	8	9	10

Not at all confident   Very confident

Comments: _____

From *The Brain Injury Rehabilitation Workbook*, edited by Rachel Winson, Barbara A. Wilson, and Andrew Bateman. Copyright © 2017 The Guilford Press. Permission to photocopy this handout is granted to purchasers of this book for personal use or for use with individual clients (see copyright page for details). Purchasers can download additional copies of this handout (see the box at the end of the table of contents).

Neurons

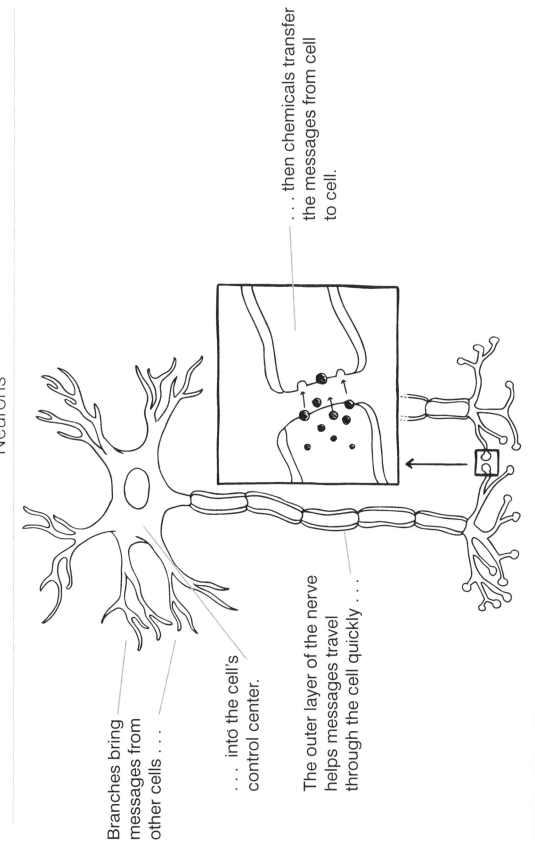

Branches bring messages from other cells . . .

. . . into the cell's control center.

The outer layer of the nerve helps messages travel through the cell quickly . . . .

. . . then chemicals transfer the messages from cell to cell.

From *The Brain Injury Rehabilitation Workbook*, edited by Rachel Winson, Barbara A. Wilson, and Andrew Bateman. Copyright © 2017 The Guilford Press. Permission to photocopy this handout is granted to purchasers of this book for personal use or for use with individual clients (see copyright page for details). Purchasers can download additional copies of this handout (see the box at the end of the table of contents).

Protection for the Brain

The skull protects the brain, though its inside surface is rough.

A fluid-filled space acts as a shock absorber.

Three membranes also support and protect the brain.

The brain has a good blood supply.

From *The Brain Injury Rehabilitation Workbook*, edited by Rachel Winson, Barbara A. Wilson, and Andrew Bateman. Copyright © 2017 The Guilford Press. Permission to photocopy this handout is granted to purchasers of this book for personal use or for use with individual clients (see copyright page for details). Purchasers can download additional copies of this handout (see the box at the er d of the table of contents).

Brain Regions

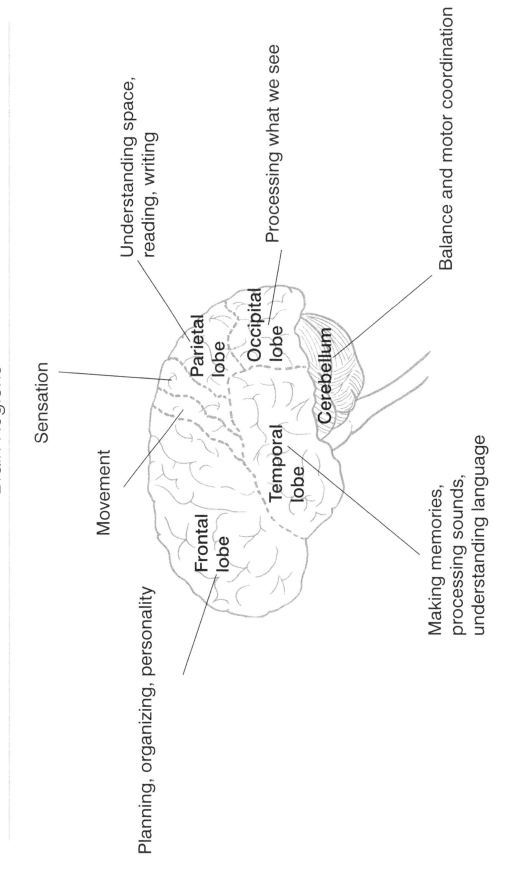

Planning, organizing, personality

Sensation

Understanding space, reading, writing

Movement

Processing what we see

Parietal lobe

Occipital lobe

Cerebellum

Balance and motor coordination

Frontal lobe

Temporal lobe

Making memories, processing sounds, understanding language

From *The Brain Injury Rehabilitation Workbook*, edited by Rachel Winson, Barbara A. Wilson, and Andrew Bateman. Copyright © 2017 The Guilford Press. Permission to photocopy this handout is granted to purchasers of this book for personal use or for use with individual clients (see copyright page for details). Purchasers can download additional copies of this handout (see the box at the end of the table of contents).

The Brain's Blood Supply

Brain seen from below

Brain cells need blood to work properly.

A dense network of blood vessels supplies blood to all parts of the brain:

- to keep it well supplied with oxygen and nutrients
- to take away toxic waste

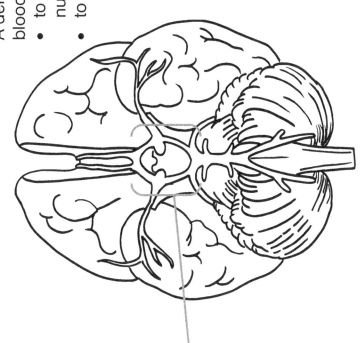

This ring of vessels allows blood to keep circulating around the brain even if one of the main arteries is blocked.

33

From *The Brain Injury Rehabilitation Workbook*, edited by Rachel Winson, Barbara A. Wilson, and Andrew Bateman. Copyright © 2017 The Guilford Press. Permission to photocopy this handout is granted to purchasers of this book for personal use or for use with individual clients (see copyright page for details). Purchasers can download additional copies of this handout (see the box at the end of the table of contents).

Understanding Brain Injury: Starting a Portfolio

Before the event that resulted in your injury:

- What were you doing? _____

    _____

- Where were you? _____

    _____

The event:

- What happened? _____

    _____

After the event:

- What type of injury did you have (traumatic brain injury, stroke, etc.)? _____

    _____

- Which areas of your brain were damaged, and how were they damaged? Use Handout 2.4 to

    help you. _____

    _____

- What happened to you while you were in the hospital (operations, monitoring, procedures,

    etc.)? _____

    _____

- How long were you in the hospital? _____

- What was your Glasgow Coma Scale score, length of coma, and length of PTA (if relevant)?

    What does this all indicate? _____

    _____

(continued)

From *The Brain Injury Rehabilitation Workbook,* edited by Rachel Winson, Barbara A. Wilson, and Andrew Bateman. Copyright © 2017 The Guilford Press. Permission to photocopy this handout is granted to purchasers of this book for personal use or for use with individual clients (see copyright page for details). Purchasers can download additional copies of this handout (see the box at the end of the table of contents).

Recovery:

- What interventions have you had since your injury (inpatient rehabilitation, outpatient therapy, etc.)? _____

  _____

- What difficulties have you experienced since the event? What support strategies have you learned? _____

  _____

Questions you have about your brain injury: _____

_____

_____

_____

_____

_____

_____

_____

_____

_____

_____

_____

_____

_____

_____

_____

_____

_____

_____

_____

CHAPTER 3

Attention

Jessica Fish
Kathrin Hicks
Susan Brentnall

One of the first psychologists who systematically investigated attention was William James. The definition of attention that he wrote in 1890 remains relevant today:

> Everyone knows what attention is. It is the taking possession by the mind, in clear and vivid form, of one out of what seems several simultaneously possible objects or trains of thought. . . . It implies withdrawal from some things in order to deal effectively with others. (James, 1890, pp. 403–404)

This chapter aims to explain the different aspects of attention, and offers a range of activities to help clients explore their own abilities and practice rehabilitation strategies.

THEORETICAL BACKGROUND, MODELS, AND NEUROANATOMY

Posner and Petersen (1990) described a framework for understanding human attention, which has been hugely influential in the field. This framework was updated in 2012 to take into account the large amount of neuroimaging research that had been conducted in the intervening period (Petersen & Posner, 2012).

The original framework set out that attention is anatomically separate from other cognitive systems (e.g., those dealing with perception or decision making), and that "attention" actually comprises three different cognitive functions across a network of brain areas. The three attention systems are as follows:

1. *The alerting system.* This system maintains a sense of "readiness to respond." It is variously referred to as "arousal," "sustained attention," or "vigilance." A degree of alertness is required in all waking situations, but examples of tasks demanding particular alertness include waiting for your order number to be called out in a café, or for your name to be called in a waiting room. Various factors affect alertness, such as task engagement, sleep deprivation, and alcohol or other substance use, and alertness naturally varies throughout the day. The alerting network includes the brain stem, reticular formation, and thalamus, and is largely right-hemisphere-lateralized (Petersen & Posner, 2012; Sturm & Wilmes, 2001). This network is illustrated in Figure 3.1, and a version of this illustration with simplified labels for clients' use is provided as Handout 3.1.*

2. *The orienting system.* This system is all about prioritizing information across the different sensory modalities (e.g., hearing, vision, touch) and across space. It is often also referred to as "selective attention." An everyday example is identifying the display board at the railway station that refers to your train, keeping your attention vaguely oriented to that location, and noticing whether the information changes. The orienting network includes areas in the frontal lobe (particularly those involved in making eye movements), the parietal lobe, and the junction between the temporal and parietal lobes. This network is illustrated in Figure 3.2, and a version of this illustration for clients' use is provided as Handout 3.2. The alerting and orienting systems work very closely together.

3. *The executive system.* As our attention is not unlimited, we need a process to control where it is directed. Ideally, this direction should be the one that is most likely to lead us toward our goals. Petersen and Posner (2012) state that there are two networks involved in this process—one for "setting up" a task according to its instructions (to continue with the example above, looking for your train on the railway station's display board), and another for

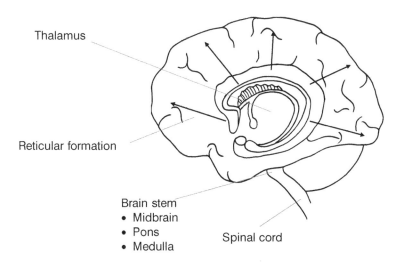

FIGURE 3.1. Brain areas involved in attention: The alerting system.

---

*All handouts are at the end of the chapter.

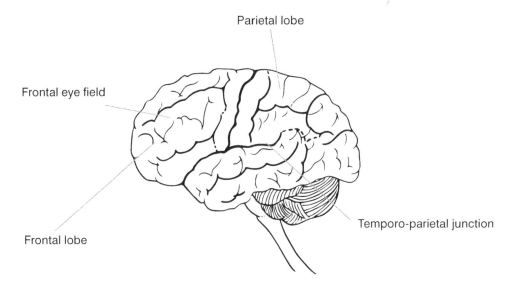

FIGURE 3.2. Brain areas involved in attention: The orienting system.

maintaining focus on that task (e.g., continuing to look for your train on the display board). When we really attend to something, this has a corresponding effect on other aspects of the attention system. For example, when the display is eventually updated to show the platform number for your train, your attention will be captured, and the resources available for other purposes (e.g., chatting to a travel companion) are temporarily reduced. This idea of limited capacity has led to the use of terms such as "switching attention" and "divided attention" to refer to situations in which we need to keep more than one thing in mind—whether such a situation involves shifting attention from one thing to another or completing two concurrent tasks. In such circumstances, it is important to consider the nature of the tasks we are dividing our attention between, as it can be more difficult to divide attention between tasks with strongly competing demands (e.g., simultaneously patting your head with one hand and rubbing your stomach with the other hand), compared with more distinct tasks (e.g., simultaneously driving and listening to the radio). There is a system of frontal and parietal brain areas involved in executive attention, with the medial frontal lobe, the anterior cingulate cortex, and the insula being particularly important. The executive system is depicted in Figure 3.3, and a version of this illustration for clients is provided as Handout 3.3.

It can be useful to keep this three-network model and its anatomical details in mind when we are trying to understand the attention problems of a client with a brain injury. We need to consider any reports of attention problems in everyday life in the context of what is known about the anatomy of the injury, and about the three attention systems. However, it is also important to remember that the different attention systems interact with each other and with other brain functions (see "Making the Links," on page 41).

For the purpose of helping clients understand attention in the context of everyday tasks, the terms "sustained attention," "selective attention," "divided attention," and "switching attention" are used in the following sections.

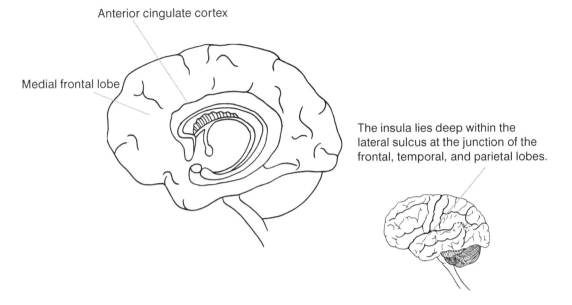

Anterior cingulate cortex

Medial frontal lobe

The insula lies deep within the lateral sulcus at the junction of the frontal, temporal, and parietal lobes.

FIGURE 3.3. Brain areas involved in attention: The executive system.

ASSESSING ATTENTION

There are various procedures for assessing aspects of attention:

- Tests of attention span, measuring how much information can be held in mind. Examples of such tests include digit span and Corsi block tests, versions of which are available in the Wechsler Adult Intelligence Scale—Fourth Edition (Wechsler, Coalson, & Raiford, 2008) and the Wechsler Memory Scale—Fourth Edition (Wechsler, Holdnack, & Drozdick, 2009).

- Tests of processing speed, measuring how quickly a person can take in and use visual or auditory information. Examples include the digit symbol and coding subtests from the Wechsler intelligence batteries, as well as the "silly sentences" test from the Speed and Capacity of Language Processing Test (Baddeley, Emslie, & Nimmo-Smith, 1992).

- Tests of vigilance/sustained attention, measuring how well a person is able to continue responding over time. Examples include the Conners Continuous Performance Test 3rd Edition (Conners, 2014) and the Sustained Attention to Response Task (Robertson, Manly, Andrade, Baddeley, & Yiend, 1997).

- Tests of more complex or executive aspects of attention, including divided attention and switching attention. Examples of such tests include trail-making and Stroop tests, versions of which are available in the Delis–Kaplan Executive Function System (Delis, Kaplan, & Kramer, 2001).

COMMON ATTENTION PROBLEMS AFTER BRAIN INJURY

Problems with attention are very common consequences of brain injury. This is not surprising, considering that attentional functions are distributed through broad neural networks. Attention problems can take different forms and have different consequences for everyday functioning, depending on the aspect(s) of attention that are affected. They can also have an impact on other domains of neuropsychological functioning, particularly memory and executive functioning (these links are explored in further detail in the next section). A thorough assessment that includes formal testing, along with functional observations and reports from clients themselves and from their caregivers, can all be helpful in understanding difficulties and designing strategies.

Some of the most common attentional difficulties are illustrated by the following case study. John was in his early 50s when he experienced a series of strokes that caused damage to his frontal and parietal lobes. The strokes had a variety of cognitive consequences, and many of them were attentional in nature. He had a strong sense that everything took longer and required more thinking power than before. On the Test of Everyday Attention (Robertson, Nimmo-Smith, Ward, & Ridgeway, 1994), his performance on all subtests was impaired relative to expectations for his age and ability. He felt that his participation in social interactions was greatly limited by this reduction; he could not keep up with conversations, or think of and contribute quips as he could before. He also had serious difficulties in tests of spatial attention; for example, his performance on the star cancellation subtest from the Behavioural Inattention Test (Wilson, Cockburn, & Halligan, 1987) was extremely slow, and he made numerous omission errors. He found environments with complex sensory inputs such as supermarkets or parties overwhelming, due to a sense of "information overload" (he felt that his senses were being bombarded). This indicated difficulties with selective attention and orienting. In addition, he had a tendency to ignore information presented on the left side of space—a spatial attention phenomenon known as "unilateral neglect." Finally, he frequently got stuck on one aspect of a situation without considering the whole, and at other times his attention would be captured by something and he would find it very difficult to go back to the original task. On the Test of Everyday Attention, he struggled particularly with the subtests of switching and divided attention. This struggle suggested a problem with executive attention.

As John's case suggests, a number of other difficulties are related to attention problems.

Reduced Speed of Processing

Speed of processing relates to the time we need to take in and respond to information—or, in other words, to how efficiently we think. People with reduced speed of processing after brain injury can have a sense that it takes more time and requires more effort to absorb information. One client at The Oliver Zangwill Centre described having a "brain like treacle" (an American client would have said, "My brain's as slow as molasses").

Distractibility

Distractibility can take various forms, depending on which aspect of attention is affected. A person may find it difficult to focus attention on a particular task or stimulus, or the person may struggle to sustain that attention over a period of time. These problems are often described in terms of difficulties with concentration. Common examples include following programs on television or the plot of a book, and blocking out irrelevant stimuli such as background noise.

Neglect

Unilateral spatial neglect involves difficulty orienting to and acting upon information from one side of space (left or right). Neglect can affect either side of space, particularly in the acute postinjury stage; later, however, it is much more likely to present as neglect of the left side of space, following right-hemisphere damage. Neglect can affect any sensory modality, although visual neglect is most common and most disabling. It can present in rather striking ways, with some people, for example, failing to dress one side of the body, comb one side of the hair, or eat from one side of the plate. There is a strong relationship between alertness and neglect (Robertson, Mattingley, Rorden, & Driver, 1998), with neglect becoming more pronounced when alertness declines, and being improved when alertness increases (e.g., through natural fluctuations and experimental manipulations such as stimulant medication).

It is important to remember that in neglect, the attentional process is impaired rather than the sensory processes, although neglect can also co-occur with visual field defects. If a client is thought to have neglect, a number of tests can be informative; these include drawing, cancellation, and bisection tasks, as well as "extinction testing" (determining whether the presence of stimuli in the intact field reduces the ability to detect stimuli in the affected field). What distinguishes between visual field loss and neglect is that people spontaneously correct for the sensory problem by turning their head and making eye movements to "fill in the gaps." People with neglect are often unaware of this missing part of space, and it is more challenging for them to remember to use such compensatory techniques.

To some extent, neglect can be overcome via the conscious direction of attention toward the neglected side. This can be achieved with the use of compensatory techniques (e.g., placing a brightly colored strip of paper at the side of the page when reading), combined with training to use those techniques (i.e., training the client to find the colored strip before they start reading each line). For a review, see Fish, Manly, and Mattingley (2012).

MAKING THE LINKS

No domain of neuropsychological functioning exists in isolation, and it is important for therapists to keep in mind the links between attention and other domains of cognitive functioning as they plan rehabilitation strategies for attention problems; memory and executive functioning are particularly linked with attention. Other factors besides cognitive domains also need to be kept in mind.

Memory

It is common for people to complain of memory problems following a brain injury when, actually, they are suffering from attention problems. What happens in such cases is that the information to be remembered is not going in properly (because of slowed processing speed, the inability to focus attention, etc.). The result is a difficulty in recalling this information, but the apparent memory problem is *caused* by one or more attentional difficulties. Formal testing can be a useful way of disentangling these processes. The observation in everyday contexts that people are far better at remembering things when strategies for improving attention are implemented (e.g., when the flow of information is slowed to a suitable pace, distractions are minimized, and prompts are given to focus and sustain attention) is also a valuable clue to the true nature of the cognitive deficit.

Executive Functioning

The demarcation between higher-level attentional processes (particularly switching and divided attention) and executive functions is somewhat hazy. Indeed, the revised Petersen and Posner (2012) model renamed "target detection" as "executive attention." Executive functions serve to organize attention, and attentional processes underpin many executive functions. It is not always practical or particularly useful in the clinic to categorize certain cognitive difficulties as involving *either* attentional *or* executive processes. But it is important to keep these links in mind, in order to help people with brain injury fully understand the nature of their difficulties and develop strategies to overcome them. (See also Winegardner, Chapter 5, this volume.)

Emotion

Emotionally salient information tends to grab our attention. Think how the attention of someone with a spider phobia is drawn not just to "creepy-crawlies" in the corner of the room, but also to things that look just a bit "spidery" or "webby," or to places where spiders have previously been found. These phenomena suggest increased alertness and orienting to this emotionally arousing information. It is also difficult to disengage attention from such stimuli (e.g., to continue working in a room with a spider would be unthinkable to a person with spider phobia), suggesting a further impact on executive attention. Many people with brain injury have a heightened sense of threat (see Ford, Chapter 8, this volume), and their attention may be preferentially drawn to any threatening information. Or they may find that the presence of "hot" (i.e., emotionally salient) goals detracts from the pursuit of other important goals, or interferes with putting "colder" cognitive strategies in place. Furthermore, difficulties with worry or rumination can consume attentional capacity and can hence mimic or exacerbate difficulties with attention. Understanding such links between cognition and emotion is an important part of a person's formulation, as once the links are made, strategies aimed at either strengthening or weakening them (as appropriate) can be devised.

Other Factors Affecting Attention

Attention is affected by a number of other factors that also have an impact on other domains of neuropsychological functioning, and these factors too must be considered in the process of assessing difficulties and planning interventions. They include the following:

- Physical factors (fatigue, pain, hunger, illness).
- Environmental factors, such as noise (auditory stimuli), clutter (visual stimuli), other people, and temperature.
- Psychological factors (anxiety, stress, anger, depression).

REHABILITATION: THE EVIDENCE

In 2014, an international group of experts (known as INCOG) published findings from a review of clinical guidelines and the published literature, to generate an authoritative set of clinical recommendations on cognitive rehabilitation after head trauma (Ponsford et al., 2014). Their primary recommendation in the domain of attention was for metacognitive strategy training, applied to personally and functionally relevant tasks (see the case studies at the end of this chapter and of Chapters 4–8 for examples of this type of training in practice). There is also evidence that training dual-tasking abilities can be effective at improving performance on those trained tasks. Therefore, if a person encounters dual-tasking difficulties in everyday life, training on the actual tasks would be advisable. Cognitive-behavioral therapy to address interactions between emotion and attention has been suggested as a potentially beneficial approach, but as there has only been one trial of this approach, further research is needed. Similarly, treatment of sleep disorders that may exacerbate attentional difficulties is also advisable. Though there is no specific guidance on what form such treatments should take, treatment trials of CBT for insomnia in people with brain injury are in progress.

Although environmental adaptations have long been recommended, there have been no formal studies of how effective they are. Given the very obvious fact that attention is a limited-capacity system, however, the principle of minimizing attentional demands via environmental adaptation seems eminently reasonable. Furthermore, the effectiveness of such strategies may be evaluated on an individual-case basis. Training on computerized tests of attention is not recommended, due to the mixed nature of the evidence from the trials that have been conducted, and the lack of any evidence for improvement following training on functional tasks. The drug methylphenidate has also been demonstrated to be effective in the short term, although data on its longer-term use are needed.

EXPLORING ATTENTION AND ITS PROBLEMS WITH CLIENTS

In order to get around the difficulties caused by our clients' attention problems, we therapists need to help the clients start noticing when the problems occur, so that together we can identify the right monitoring strategies to use. A monitoring sheet is provided as Handout

3.4 for you to support your clients in developing self-awareness; getting feedback from others can also support clients' increased awareness of the frequency and nature of attention slips. Video-recording clients (with their consent) while they perform functional tasks, and reviewing the footage later, can be another useful way of raising awareness.

What Is Attention?

Before introducing the activities and strategies, you will probably find it helpful to do some basic psychoeducation with clients, looking at different types of attention, the ways the brain works in these different types, and some common difficulties. This can help the clients to start considering their own strengths and challenges. Use Handouts 3.5 and 3.6 to help clients understand the different aspects of attention.

What Can Happen to Attention after Brain Injury?

Handout 3.7 offers some real-life examples from clients of how it feels to have attention problems. Ask your clients whether any of these difficulties resonate with them. Handout 3.8 gives an illustration of some external and internal factors that can be distracting. Ask clients to identify possible distractions in the picture. Another way of exploring the importance of attention in everyday life is to get clients to complete driving hazard perception tests, some of which are available free of charge online.

Helping Clients Explore Their Attentional Abilities

This section suggests some activities to help clients explore their own abilities. Some clients may find it helpful if you contextualize the tasks by relating the skills being explored to everyday tasks; suggestions for doing this are provided in the bullet points on pages 45 and 46. Support clients in reflecting on the experience: What was easy? What was difficult? Were they able to notice when their attention was slipping? The activities can be repeated to trial the strategies outlined. Again, offer feedback and support clients to reflect on how well the strategies worked for them.

   If the tasks are too simple for some clients, you can increase the challenge by introducing background noise, interruptions, or visual distractions such as a cluttered environment. For clients who are struggling, aim to minimize visual and auditory distractions.

   To practice *sustained auditory attention*, clients can listen to radio clips such as extended weather forecasts, news reports, or football scores, all of which can be sourced from Internet radio players. Ask clients to listen for key pieces of information. Consider whether the task is easier if the subject matter is of interest to a client; for example, does someone who is interested in football find it easier to focus on the scores than, say, the weather forecast? Also ask the clients to recall other details, because often they are so intent on listening for the target information that they don't attend to the rest of the content. Discuss this with them and ask them to think of how this might interfere with their functioning in day-to-day life. Then encourage clients to try the task again, using an appropriate strategy (e.g., the attention beam, managing external distractions; see the discussion of strategies on pages 45 and 46).

- Related everyday situations: watching a film/TV program; listening to a lecture; listening for a particular region to be mentioned in a weather report.

To explore *selective visual attention*, ask clients how many animals they can find in the image on Handout 3.9, within a time limit (the answer is 12, although remember the answer isn't that important; it's the process that counts!). To practice using scanning or the attention beam, ask them to find a particular item in the photo in Handout 3.10.

- Related everyday situations: finding the right brand of toothpaste on a supermarket shelf; locating an item in a crowded drawer; searching for a friend in a crowd.

The following activity explores *auditory selective attention*. With a colleague, read two newspaper articles aloud at the same time; alternatively, play two different radio news broadcasts simultaneously, or for an even greater challenge, play a TV news clip alongside a radio broadcast. Then ask questions about one of the articles or clips to determine whether clients could focus their attention. Did they pick up any details from the second article or clip? Then try the task again, encouraging clients to use the attention beam to focus.

- Related everyday situations: listening to a conversation with background noise in a busy restaurant; talking on the telephone at work when the office is busy; screening out the radio, TV, or music when a client's children are both talking to the client at the same time.

To practice *switching attention*, give clients copies of a word search, a crossword, and a Sudoku sourced from puzzle magazines. Explain that you are going to ask them to begin one of the puzzles, then to switch to the next. Either set a timer, or tap the table after about 30 seconds have passed to cue the change. Repeat this process several times. What did clients notice? Common difficulties might include taking a while to get going with each new task, perseveration, difficulty recalling the overarching instruction once they were absorbed in a puzzle, and/or difficulty picking up where they left off when returning to a task. Then try a second set of activities, using a strategy. For example, ask clients to use Stop/Think (see Winegardner, Chapter 5, this volume) to consciously halt their train of thought and switch their focus to the new task in hand.

- Related everyday situations: breaking off from working on the computer to answer a phone call; having to stop in the middle of cooking a meal to answer the door; having a conversation interrupted by a question from someone else.

Next, explore *divided attention*. Make sure clients understand the difference between switching attention (moving attention from one task to another) and divided attention (focusing on more than one task at the same time). Then ask them to complete a word search, Sudoku, crossword, or connect-the-dots puzzle while listening to you asking them questions about themselves. Did they notice themselves dividing or switching their attention? Next, ask clients to complete the puzzle while listing as many words as possible beginning with the letter D. What do they notice? Clients may also like to try two motor tasks at the same time (e.g., patting their heads while rubbing their stomachs) or a cognitive and a motor task together (e.g., naming musical instruments while walking). Do they find certain combinations of tasks harder than others, and are they even aware when they are doing two or more things at the same time? Help clients to consider whether one task needs more effort or is easier than the other. Do they stay on track and successfully complete both tasks, or are they just ignoring one and concentrating on the other?

If clients are aware of which combinations are harder for them, advise them to practice tasks to make them more automatic, allowing them to focus most attention on the hardest task. They can also use the attention beam to switch their attention frequently between the tasks.

- Related everyday situations: walking and talking at the same time; driving while listening to the radio; eating while watching TV.

The images provided in Handout 3.11 can help clients explore their abilities with regard to visuospatial attention in general. You can place the pictures provided in this handout on the walls along a corridor (about five on each side) and ask the clients to walk along the corridor; alternatively, you can spread the pictures in a semicircle in front of the clients. Ask what they see. The activity can then be repeated, using the lighthouse strategy described on page 47. Did clients notice more pictures this time?

- Related everyday situations: searching a webpage for information; scanning supermarket shelves, cupboards, or bookshelves; avoiding obstacles in the street; noticing which shops in a shopping center or mall have sales going on; noticing information signs about changes to class times at a local gym or sports center.

REHABILITATION STRATEGIES

Attention Beam

The "attention beam" strategy involves focusing on some things while ignoring others—much as when we use a flashlight in a darkened room. The flashlight beam illuminates the object we're shining it on, while leaving the rest of the room in darkness. We can all think of our attention as being like a flashlight beam. Sometimes we need to move our attention from place to place, just as a flashlight beam can be shone on different corners of a room. Encourage clients to personalize the strategy: Some might prefer to think of the beam as a miner's lamp, a spotlight, a car headlight, or a searchlight. When clients are doing tasks that involve switching or dividing attention, they can envision using more than one attention beam.

There is some evidence that attention can be improved through repetitive practice. However, it is important that the tasks used in training are functionally relevant, as there is little evidence that gains made during training generalize to untrained tasks. See Evans, Greenfield, Wilson, and Bateman (2009).

Lighthouse

The "lighthouse" strategy is an extension of the attention beam strategy to support scanning. It can be particularly helpful with clients experiencing visuospatial attention problems (such problems can be manifested in everyday life as bumping into or tripping over things, struggling to find items on supermarket shelves, or hunting for things in drawers or cupboards at home). Using the lighthouse strategy can help clients consciously direct their attention to both sides of space.

Show the clients a simple diagram of a lighthouse. Tell them that their eyes are like the lights inside the top, sweeping all the way to the left and right of the horizon to guide the ships at sea to safety. Ask, "What would happen if the lighthouse lit only the right or left side of the ocean and the horizon?" Demonstrate turning your head from side to side to allow your eyes to sweep left and right like a lighthouse beam. Align the tip of the chin with the top of the right shoulder, then move the head slowly around so that the chin is in line with the top of the left shoulder. Emphasize the importance of the physical movement, as this increases alertness, and, as stated previously, there is a strong link between alertness and spatial attention.

Reducing External Distractions

Handout 3.8 can be used again to identify external distractions. Now ask clients to consider how these might best be managed. Here are some suggestions for clients to try.

- Reduce background noise: Turn off the TV, radio, music, heater, and other electrical equipment, and close the window to screen out traffic noise.
- Complete important or difficult tasks in a quiet room if possible.
- Switch off mobile phones, turn down the volume on the landline, and let an answering machine or voicemail take messages.
- Switch off automatic email notifications.
- Use ear plugs if necessary. Noise-canceling headphones can also be extremely effective for clients experiencing hyperacusis, or sensitivity to noise, after brain injury.
- Reduce visual distractions: Declutter! Sit at a cleared-off table with just the items needed to complete the task in hand. Try not to sit opposite a window, as this can create distractions. Conversely, some people find looking at a bare wall distracting so it can help to try out different approaches and identify the space that works best for you.
- Make sure the lighting in the workspace is adequate.

Reducing Internal Distractions

As noted earlier, attention can be affected by internal sensations as well as external distractors. Thoughts, feelings, and physical sensations such as pain may distract clients from focusing on tasks. Ask clients to practice focusing on a single spot or closing the eyes for 2 minutes. Then ask clients to notice whether their attention wandered. What physical sensations did they have? What thoughts came into their heads? Next, review the attention beam strategy, and explain that the clients are going to practice turning the beam inward to notice when they're being distracted. When the beam is directed toward a thought or sensation, encourage clients to notice, and gently direct their attention back to the central focal point. Clients may also wish to explore the mood management strategies outlined by Ford in Chapter 8, which can help to reduce internal distractions.

Managing Visual Attention Difficulties

If clients experience neglect, encourage them to place objects or other targets to be perceived on their "good" side. Visuospatial neglect can be problematic when clients are reading; they can use a finger, ruler, or marker to bring them back to the start of a line. Route finding can also be challenging for people with visual attention problems. They may find it helpful to use landmarks, satellite navigation systems, maps, and signposts to find the way, rather than relying on their sense of direction. Simple routes can also be practiced by means of "errorless learning" (in which clients are shown the correct sequences of a step-by-step route, without the opportunity to make mistakes, and then supported to gradually take on more responsibility for navigating some of the steps, when they are sure that they know the correct direction in which to proceed, until the route can be independently reproduced).

BRINGING IT ALL TOGETHER

Once clients have learned more about their own attention profiles and identified some strategies they would like to try, the following functional activities can be used to practice strategies. A behavioral experiment approach (described in more detail by Winegardner, Chapter 5, and Ford, Chapter 8, this volume) can be used to explore clients' beliefs about their abilities. Some possible experiments include the following:

- Cooking a multicomponent meal. Clients can experiment within their home environment to see what works best for them. Perhaps switching off the radio, closing the door, clearing the work surfaces of all but essential items, or temporarily banishing the rest of the family from the kitchen might help. Ask clients how cooking in a real-life family environment feels, as compared to preparing a meal in an assessment setting.

- Supermarket shopping with instructions to buy specific items. This can be tried in two ways—first with you or a family member chatting throughout, and then without the disruption of conversation. Afterward, get the clients to compare how effectively they performed each time and how the experience felt.

- Visiting a library, art gallery, museum, or exhibition, with a view to locating specific pieces of information by using either visual displays or audio guides.

- Completing a local treasure hunt (obtainable through the Internet). This can be an enjoyable way of practicing attention strategies in the community. Other needs, such as overcoming social anxiety and practicing communication skills, can also be addressed in this context.

- Watching a film/TV program with discussion afterward. This can also be tried in two ways—alone in a quiet room, and in a typical family setting with distractions. Clients can compare how much they got from the program in each case, and whether the environment made the task any more enjoyable or less tiring.

- Assembling a piece of furniture from a kit, using audio, video, or written instructions. As with the cooking task described above, clients can try completing this or other do-it-yourself tasks in different environments.

- Holding a conversation, doing a quiz, or completing a crossword in a noisy café.

- Reading a newspaper on a busy train platform while keeping an eye on the train departure time.

- Using a bus or train timetable to plan a journey.

- Phoning a local cinema and listening to recorded information to find when a particular film is showing.

- Finding specific information on a website (e.g., a site offering used car ads or financial advice; such sites are usually crammed with information).

COMPLETING AN ATTENTION PROFILE

Clients may wish to complete a copy of the attention profile sheet (Handout 3.12) to add to their portfolios. Use the information gathered from monitoring sheets and activities to help clients identify their strengths and challenges with regard to attention.

CASE STUDY

In practice, it is difficult for therapists to separate attention, memory, and executive functioning when working to implement strategies for any area with clients in therapy. The following case study covers both areas of cognitive functioning.

Jeff sustained a severe traumatic brain injury in a road traffic accident at the age of 19. Prior to his injury, he had been a promising golfer who was preparing to take up a sports scholarship in the United States. After his accident, despite recovering well from his physical injuries, he struggled to resume work and study because of his significant cognitive difficulties. The problems Jeff faced with regard to attention and memory, and some of his goals and strategies for dealing with these problems, are described in Table 3.1.

TABLE 3.1. Dealing with Jeff's Attention and Memory Challenges

Challenges	Goals and strategies	Context for rehabilitation
Impaired divided attention Jeff enjoyed cooking, but frequently spoiled meals because he became distracted in the kitchen. *Working memory—low average* Jeff struggled to keep the instructions in mind while following multistep recipes. He also frequently forgot items when doing his grocery shopping. *Impaired verbal and nonverbal recognition memory; slow, inefficient verbal learning* Jeff was keen to broaden his culinary repertoire, but found it difficult to learn new recipes. Prior to his injury, Jeff's memory had been good, and he had never needed to rely on memory aids. He was understandably reluctant to try strategies in the first instance.	Goals: To learn new recipes that could be cooked at home for the family. Compensatory strategies: • Personal organizer alerts and reminders • Stop/Think (see Chapter 5) • Goal Management Framework (GMF; see Chapter 5) • Environmental adaptation Behavioral experiments to challenge Jeff's negative beliefs about the use of memory aids.	Jeff was supported to plan, shop for, and cook a meal for staff and fellow clients. Jeff created a lunch invitation to circulate around the center, using Stop/Think to check that he had included all the key details. He also made a questionnaire to check out special dietary needs. Jeff identified a new recipe that he wanted to try, using the GMF to weigh his options. With help, he broke the recipe down into simple steps that he rewrote in his own words in the form of a checklist. This checklist was laminated and tested in a practice cooking session to build Jeff's confidence. During this session, Jeff learned that reducing clutter in the kitchen and turning off the radio helped him focus while cooking. Jeff was helped to use his personal organizer as a planning tool. He wrote a shopping list, checking which ingredients were already available in the therapy kitchen; created a timeline for the day; and recorded his expenditures. Mobile phone alerts were used to remind Jeff to go to the supermarket for ingredients—and to bring them in on the right day! He also used the timer on his phone to keep him on track while cooking.

REFERENCES

Baddeley, A., Emslie, H., & Nimmo-Smith, I. (1992). *Speed and Capacity of Language Processing Test (SCOLP) reference materials.* London: Pearson.

Conners, C. K. (2014). *Conners Continuous Performance Test 3rd Edition (CPT 3).* North Tonawanda, NY: Multi-Health Systems.

Delis, D. C., Kaplan, E., & Kramer, J. H. (2001). *Delis–Kaplan Executive Function System (D-KEFS).* London: Pearson.

Evans, J. J., Greenfield, E., Wilson, B. A., & Bateman, A. (2009). Walking and talking therapy: Improving cognitive–motor dual-tasking in neurological illness. *Journal of the International Society: JINS, 15*(1), 112–120.

James, W. (1890). *The principles of psychology.* New York: Holt.

Manly, T., Fish, J., & Mattingley, J. (2012). Visuospatial and attentional disorders. In L. H. Goldstein & J. E. McNeil (Eds.), *Clinical neuropsychology: A practical guide to assessment and management for clinicians* (2nd ed., pp. 261–291). Chichester, UK: Wiley.

Petersen, S. E., & Posner, M. I. (2012). The attention system of the human brain: 20 years after. *Annual Review of Neuroscience, 35,* 73–89.

Ponsford, J., Bayley, M., Wiseman-Hakes, C., Togher, L., Velikonja, D., McIntyre, A., et al. (2014). INCOG recommendations for management of cognition following traumatic brain injury: Part II. Attention and information processing speed. *Journal of Head Trauma Rehabilitation, 29*(4), 321–337.

Posner, M. I., & Petersen, S. E. (1990). The attention system of the human brain. *Annual Review of Neuroscience, 13,* 25–42.

Robertson, I. H., Manly, T., Andrade, J., Baddeley, B. T., & Yiend, J. (1997). 'Oops!': Performance correlates of everyday attentional failures in traumatic brain injured and normal subjects. *Neuropsychologia, 35,* 747–758.

Robertson, I. H., Mattingley, J. B., Rorden, C., & Driver, J. (1998). Phasic alerting of neglect patients overcomes their spatial deficit in visual awareness. *Nature, 395*(6698), 169–172.

Robertson, I. H., Nimmo-Smith, I., Ward, T., & Ridgeway, V. (1994). *The Test of Everday Attention (YEA).* London: Pearson Clinical.

Sturm, W., & Wilmes, K. (2001). On the functional neuroanatomy of intrinsic and phasic alertness. *NeuroImage, 14,* S76–S84.

Wechsler, D., Coalson, D. L., & Raiford, S. E. (2008). *Wechsler Adult Intelligence Scale—Fourth Edition: Technical and interpretive manual.* San Antonio, TX: Pearson.

Wechsler, D., Holdnack, J. A., & Drozdick, L. W. (2009). *Wechsler Memory Scale—Fourth Edition: Technical and interpretive manual.* San Antonio, TX: Pearson.

Wilson, B. A., Cockburn, J., & Halligan, P. W. (1987). *The Behavioural Inattention Test.* London: Pearson Clinical.

Brain Areas Involved in Attention: The Alerting System

Parts of the "old brain" filter information from our senses . . .

. . . and a network of nerve fibers passes it on to the rest of the brain.

Brain stem

The spinal cord brings information from our senses.

These parts of the brain are involved in staying alert and getting ready to respond:

- listening for your name to be called at the dentist's office
- looking out for the platform of your train on the station departure board
- waiting in line for your order number to be called at a café

From *The Brain Injury Rehabilitation Workbook*, edited by Rachel Winson, Barbara A. Wilson, and Andrew Bateman. Copyright © 2017 The Guilford Press. Permission to photocopy this handout is granted to purchasers of this book for personal use or for use with individual clients (see copyright page for details). Purchasers can download additional copies of this handout (see the box at the end of the table of contents).

Brain Areas Involved in Attention: The Orienting System

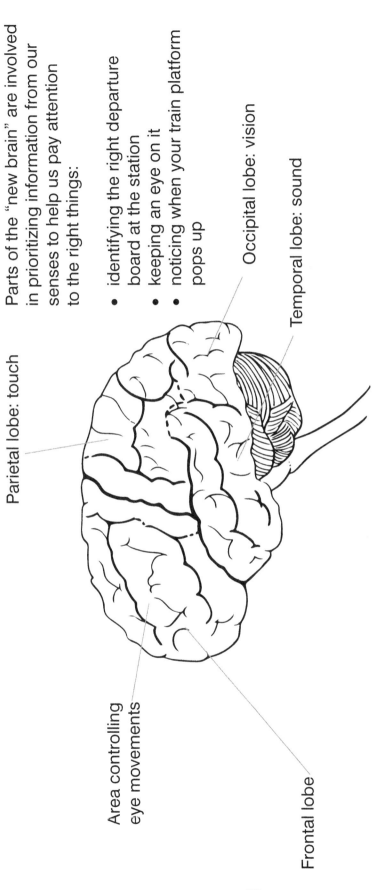

Parietal lobe: touch

Parts of the "new brain" are involved in prioritizing information from our senses to help us pay attention to the right things:

- identifying the right departure board at the station
- keeping an eye on it
- noticing when your train platform pops up

Occipital lobe: vision

Temporal lobe: sound

Area controlling eye movements

Frontal lobe

The "new brain" and "old brain" work closely together when we are paying attention to something.

From *The Brain Injury Rehabilitation Workbook*, edited by Rachel Winson, Barbara A. Wilson, and Andrew Bateman. Copyright © 2017 The Guilford Press. Permission to photocopy this handout is granted to purchasers of this book for personal use or for use with individual clients (see copyright page for details). Purchasers can download additional copies of this handout (see the box at the end of the table of contents).

Brain Areas Involved in Attention: The Executive System

These parts of the brain are involved in controlling our attention so that we meet our goals.

Sometimes we need to pay attention to two things at once (e.g., walking and talking).

Sometimes we need to move our attention quickly from one thing to another (e.g., if the phone rings while we are working).

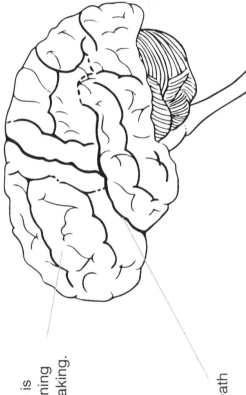

The frontal lobe is involved in planning and decision making.

The insula lies underneath the brain's surface. It monitors internal states and emotions.

From *The Brain Injury Rehabilitation Workbook*, edited by Rachel Winson, Barbara A. Wilson, and Andrew Bateman. Copyright © 2017 The Guilford Press. Permission to photocopy this handout is granted to purchasers of this book for personal use or for use with individual clients (see copyright page for details). Purchasers can download additional copies of this handout (see the box at the end of the table of contents).

Attention Monitoring

Date/time	What were you doing? What happened?	What was the environment like?	How were you feeling?

From *The Brain Injury Rehabilitation Workbook*, edited by Rachel Winson, Barbara A. Wilson, and Andrew Bateman. Copyright © 2017 The Guilford Press. Permission to photocopy this handout is granted to purchasers of this book for personal use or for use with individual clients (see copyright page for details). Purchasers can download additional copies of this handout (see the box at the end of the table of contents).

Sustained versus Selective Attention

Sustained Attention

- Staying focused on what you're doing, even if it's not that interesting.
- Concentrating! Sustained attention can be visual (looking/watching) or auditory (listening).

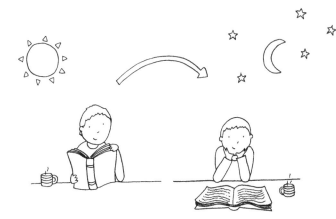

When do you use it?

Listening to a lecture/class at school.

Driving on a long journey.

Listening to the radio.

Reading a book or newspaper.

Watching a film or TV program.

Selective Attention

- Ignoring or filtering out distractions, so you can concentrate on what is important.

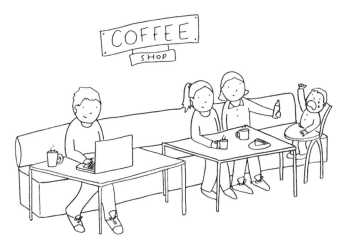

When do you use it?

Picking out the information you need from a busy webpage.

Talking on your cell phone on a street with lots of traffic going past.

Using a laptop in a coffee shop when a baby is crying at the next table.

Listening to a whole weather report to hear the forecast for your area.

Listening to someone talk in a crowded restaurant.

Crossing the road safely.

Finding your brand of coffee on the supermarket shelf.

From *The Brain Injury Rehabilitation Workbook*, edited by Rachel Winson, Barbara A. Wilson, and Andrew Bateman. Copyright © 2017 The Guilford Press. Permission to photocopy this handout is granted to purchasers of this book for personal use or for use with individual clients (see copyright page for details). Purchasers can download additional copies of this handout (see the box at the end of the table of contents).

Switching Attention versus Divided Attention

Switching Attention

- Moving attention from one task to another when it is important to do so.

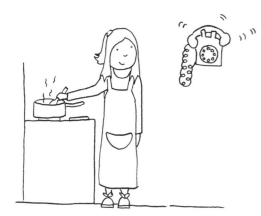

When do you use it?

Answering the phone in the middle of typing a report.

Cooking a complex meal, and realizing that a pan is about to boil over when you're in the middle of chopping other ingredients.

Driving along "on autopilot" and listening to the radio, when the traffic suddenly slows ahead and you have to brake sharply.

Divided Attention

- Concentrating on more than one thing at once.
- This is hard!

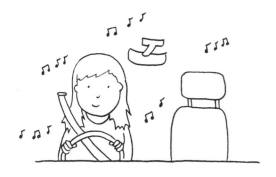

When do you use it?

Driving or working and listening to the radio.

Walking and talking.

Drinking a coffee while walking down the street.

From *The Brain Injury Rehabilitation Workbook*, edited by Rachel Winson, Barbara A. Wilson, and Andrew Bateman. Copyright © 2017 The Guilford Press. Permission to photocopy this handout is granted to purchasers of this book for personal use or for use with individual clients (see copyright page for details). Purchasers can download additional copies of this handout (see the box at the end of the table of contents).

How Does It Feel?

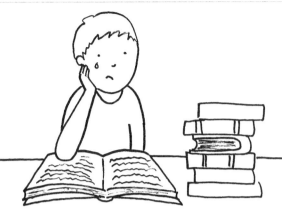

"I used to enjoy reading, but I can't do it now."

"When I'm driving with the kids in the car, I've had to tell them to be quiet, as I can't concentrate."

"I find it difficult watching television at home when my family members are doing things around me, whether they're chatting with each other or using their cell phones or computers."

"I start something and get distracted by something else. By the end of the day, I feel exhausted and don't feel I've achieved anything."

"Cooking is difficult. I'm not able to do two things at the same time, so I've started to find easier recipes where it is possible to do one step at a time."

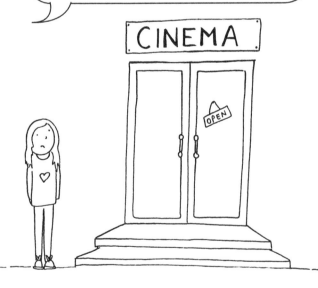

"I can't go to the cinema any more."

From *The Brain Injury Rehabilitation Workbook*, edited by Rachel Winson, Barbara A. Wilson, and Andrew Bateman. Copyright © 2017 The Guilford Press. Permission to photocopy this handout is granted to purchasers of this book for personal use or for use with individual clients (see copyright page for details). Purchasers can download additional copies of this handout (see the box at the end of the table of contents).

Environmental Distractions

Which of the things in the picture might affect your ability to pay attention?

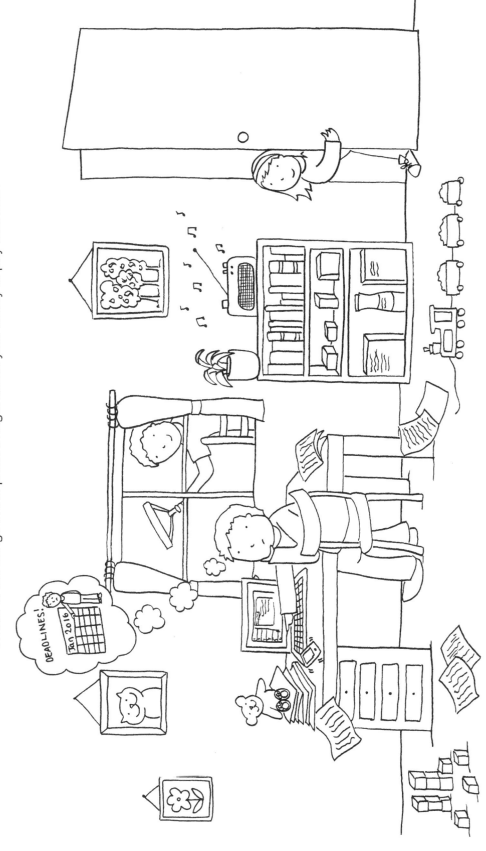

From *The Brain Injury Rehabilitation Workbook*, edited by Rachel Winson, Barbara A. Wilson, and Andrew Bateman. Copyright © 2017 The Guilford Press. Permission to photocopy this handout is granted to purchasers of this book for personal use or for use with individual clients (see copyright page for details). Purchasers can download additional copies of this handout (see the box at the end of the table of contents).

Selective Visual Attention (1)

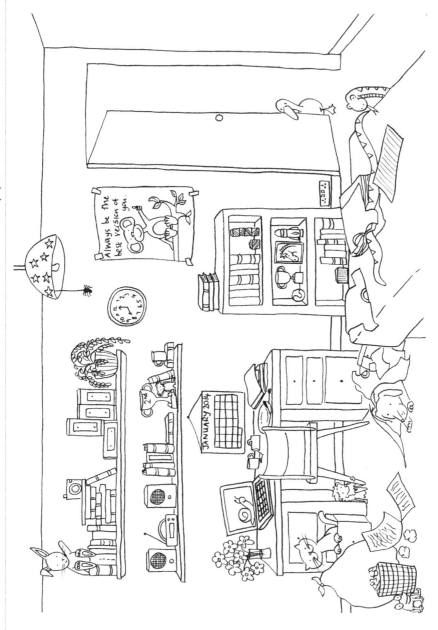

How many animals can you find in this image?

Were you aware of using any strategies? If so, what were they? If not, are there any strategies you could use?

From *The Brain Injury Rehabilitation Workbook*, edited by Rachel Winson, Barbara A. Wilson, and Andrew Bateman. Copyright © 2017 The Guilford Press. Permission to photocopy this handout is granted to purchasers of this book for personal use or for use with individual clients (see copyright page for details). Purchasers can download additional copies of this handout (see the box at the end of the table of contents).

Selective Visual Attention (2)

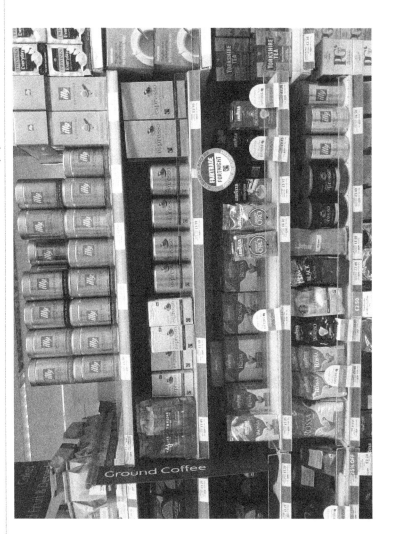

Can you find PG Tips brand of tea in this picture?

Were you aware of using any strategies? If so, what were they? If not, are there any strategies you could use?

From *The Brain Injury Rehabilitation Workbook*, edited by Rachel Winson, Barbara A. Wilson, and Andrew Bateman. Copyright © 2017 The Guilford Press. Permission to photocopy this handout is granted to purchasers of this book for personal use or for use with individual clients (see copyright page for details). Purchasers can download additional copies of this handout (see the box at the end of the table of contents).

Visuospatial Attention

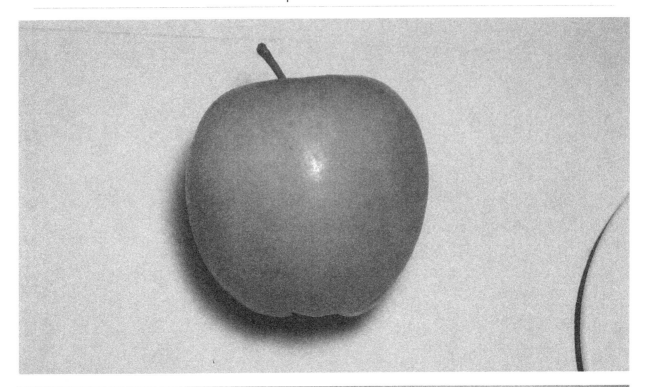

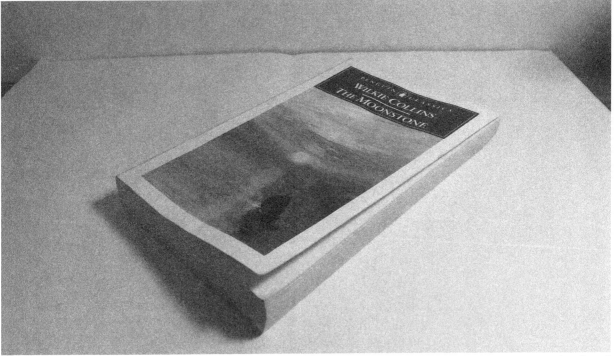

(continued)

From *The Brain Injury Rehabilitation Workbook*, edited by Rachel Winson, Barbara A. Wilson, and Andrew Bateman. Copyright © 2017 The Guilford Press. Permission to photocopy this handout is granted to purchasers of this book for personal use or for use with individual clients (see copyright page for details). Purchasers can download additional copies of this handout (see the box at the end of the table of contents).

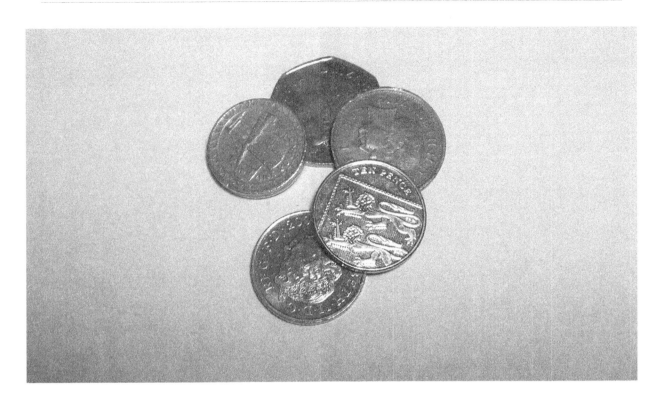

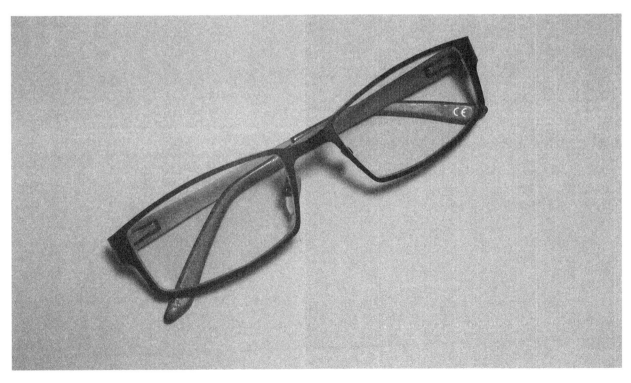

(continued)

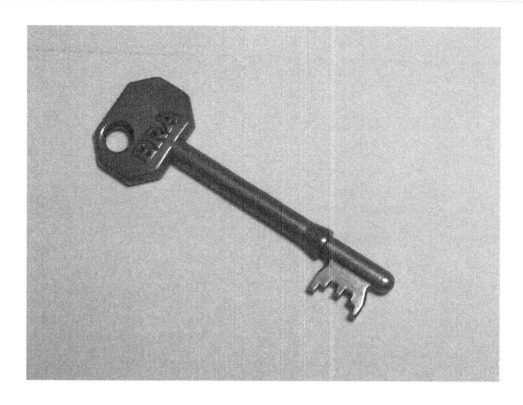

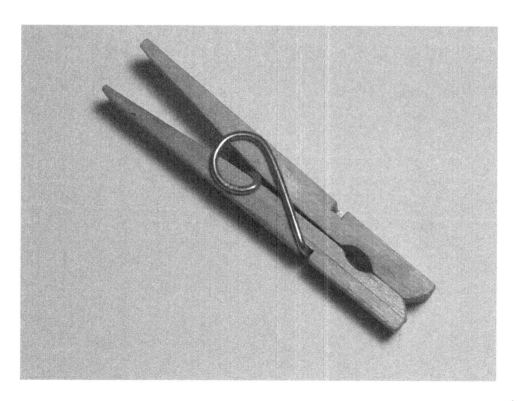

(continued)

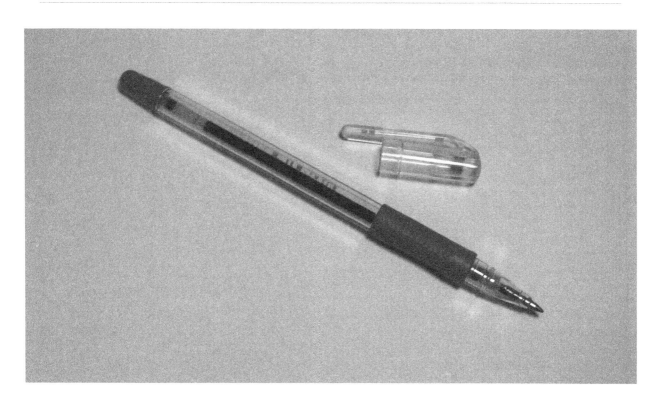

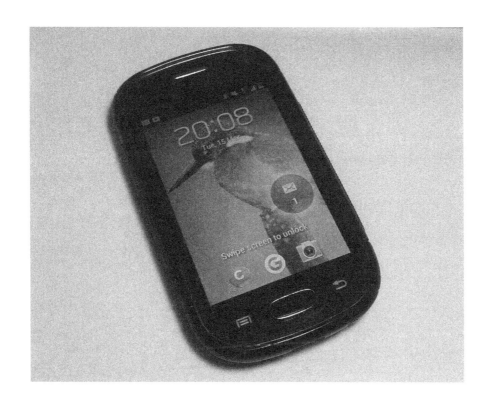

(continued)

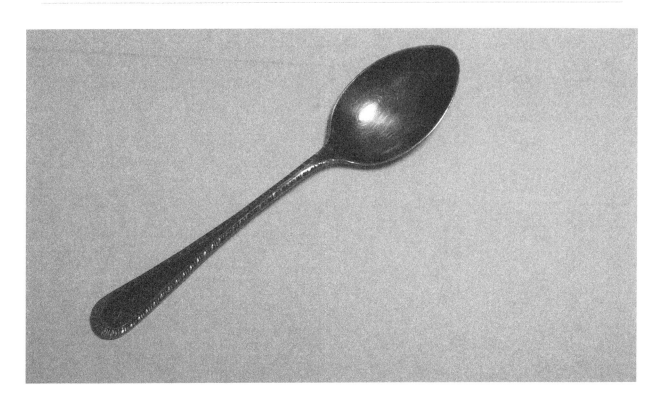

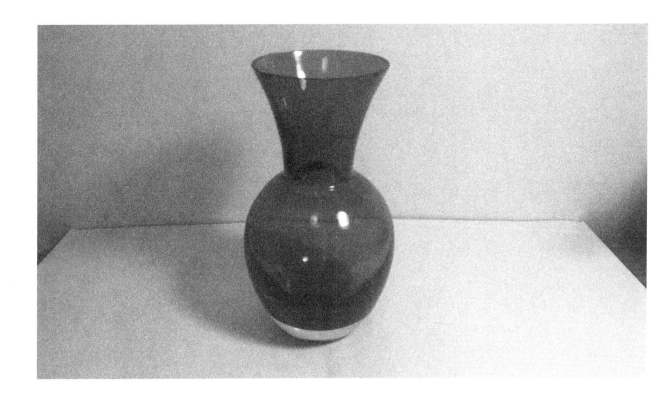

My Attention Profile

Type of attention	Strengths (with examples)	Challenges (with examples)	What makes it harder?	What makes it easier?
Sustained attention				
Selective attention				
Switching attention				
Divided attention				
Visuospatial attention				

From *The Brain Injury Rehabilitation Workbook*, edited by Rachel Winson, Barbara A. Wilson, and Andrew Bateman. Copyright © 2017 The Guilford Press. Permission to photocopy this handout is granted to purchasers of this book for personal use or for use with individual clients (see copyright page for details). Purchasers can download additional copies of this handout (see the box at the end of the table of contents).

CHAPTER 4

Memory

Jessica Fish
Susan Brentnall

When we talk casually about memory, we often tend to treat it as an all-or-nothing entity. We might describe someone as having "a memory like a sieve" to indicate poor ability to remember, or conversely as having memory like an elephant if the person seems to have particularly detailed recollections. This actually rather misrepresents what we know about memory from the last century or more of psychological study: "Memory" actually refers to a collection of processes and abilities ranging from knowing how to ride a bike, to recalling what we had for breakfast, to imagining the future. All of these abilities are used, day in and day out, in our relationships, work, activities, and chores.

This chapter sets out educational information about memory; then provides activities to use with clients to help them explore their own memory strengths and challenges, along with a range of strategies to facilitate memory. Note that these strategies will not fix or improve overall memory, but they will help clients to use their remaining memory skills and associated cognitive functions more effectively to facilitate progress toward rehabilitation goals.

These strategies are based on psychology experiments that involved multiple trials. On average, use of each strategy was associated with better performance than that produced by either no strategy or a comparison strategy. The strategies broadly apply to three areas: learning new information, remembering past events, and remembering to do things. It is worth remembering that not every strategy works for every person, and that it can be worth trying a strategy several times, whether or not the first trial was successful.

THEORETICAL BACKGROUND AND MODELS

There are two important things to know about memory:

1. There are three stages of memory: "encoding" (taking in information), "storage" (keeping some representation of that information), and "retrieval" (finding that information when it is needed). We can think of this as like a filing system—creating the original file, putting it in the right section, and finding it again when it is needed next.

2. There are several different types of memory, organized in different brain areas, and involved in different everyday tasks. The types of memory problems clients experience are likely to depend upon the parts of the brain affected by their injuries, as well as the types of activities they are involved with on a day-to-day basis.

Squire and Knowlton (1995) came up with a good way of organizing these components; a schematic diagram of this model is shown in Figure 4.1. First, there is a distinction between memory that we are aware of (called "explicit" or "declarative" memory, as we can "declare" the contents), and memory that we are unaware of ("implicit" or "nondeclarative" memory).

Implicit memory includes the following:

- *Procedural memory:* Memory for nonverbal skills and motor procedures, such as knowing how to ride a bike or play an instrument.

- *Priming:* A type of memory where we may not remember having seen or heard something before, but are quicker to learn or recognize it the second time around.

- *Conditioning:* A type of memory in which we learn to associate one thing with another without having a conscious awareness of the link. For example, in a famous

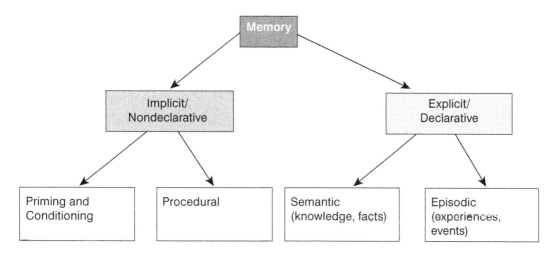

FIGURE 4.1. A schematic diagram of the Squire and Knowlton (1995) taxonomy of long-term memory.

psychology experiment, if dogs were fed alongside the sound of a bell ringing, they eventually began to salivate whenever they heard the bell ringing, indicating that they expected to receive food.

The main point about implicit memory as far as rehabilitation is concerned is that it is very rarely affected by brain injury, and so implicit memory can be used to establish new routines that can facilitate goal attainment. An example is to keep house keys in the same place to avoid losing them.

Explicit memory includes the following:

- *Episodic memory:* Our memory for events. The memory scientist Endel Tulving (2002) says that memory allows us to engage in "mental time travel," as we can conjure up recollections of the past and imagine the future.

- *Prospective memory:* Our memory for future intentions, such as remembering to buy milk on the way home. This type of memory is often a challenge for people after brain injury, as it also relies on attention and executive functioning (Fish, Wilson, & Manly, 2010).

- *Semantic memory:* Our store of information about what words mean, what objects look/sound/feel like, and facts about the world in general. Examples include knowing that a spider has eight legs without needing to count them, and that the object making a trilling noise in the hallway is called a telephone. This information is not necessarily linked with the time or place in which it was acquired. This type of memory can be damaged in some types of brain injury, particularly that involving the anterior temporal lobes (i.e., the frontmost part of the temporal lobes; Patterson, Nestor, & Rogers, 2007).

- *Working memory:* The system that holds and manipulates information currently "in mind," which was first described by Baddeley and Hitch (1974). For instance, when someone reads aloud a phone number for us, we hold the digits in mind while we dial the number or write it down.

The taxonomy described above and depicted in Figure 4.1 can help clients to understand that there is no one such thing as "memory"; rather, there are several different types of memory, which can be independently affected by brain injury. Different experiences of memory problems in day-to-day life can result, and strengths in one domain can be used to compensate for weaknesses in other areas. This can be the basis for beginning to use strategies.

NEUROANATOMY OF MEMORY

People with brain injuries have played a large role in developing our understanding of memory. Many scientific studies of memory from the 1950s to the present day have concerned different patterns of memory difficulty shown by people with damage to different brain regions, or with particular types of brain disease. Scientists have also used brain imaging

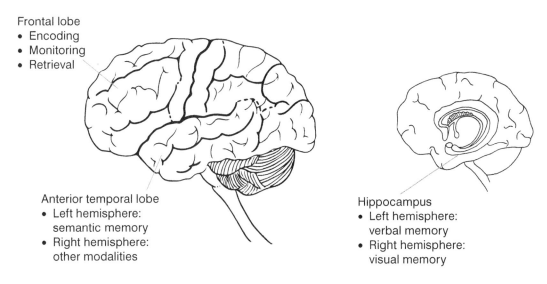

Frontal lobe
- Encoding
- Monitoring
- Retrieval

Anterior temporal lobe
- Left hemisphere: semantic memory
- Right hemisphere: other modalities

Hippocampus
- Left hemisphere: verbal memory
- Right hemisphere: visual memory

FIGURE 4.2. Brain areas involved in memory.

technologies to find out more about which areas are involved in the different types of memory, and the different processes within these types. Figure 4.2 illustrates some of the brain areas involved in different memory types and processes, and a version of this illustration with simplified labels for clients' use is provided as Handout 4.1.* The following aspects of neuroanatomy are particularly important to consider in rehabilitation:

- Episodic memory is frequently affected by brain injury, particularly that involving the medial temporal lobes. These lobes include a structure called the hippocampus, which is thought to be particularly important in learning (Squire & Zola-Morgan, 1991); the left-hemisphere portion of the hippocampus is believed to be particularly involved in verbal memory, and the right-hemisphere portion in visual memory (Kelley et al., 1998). There are also important frontal lobe contributions to episodic memory, particularly in terms of encoding, monitoring, and retrieval (Fletcher & Henson, 2001).
- The anterior temporal lobes are heavily involved in semantic memory. Again, the left lobe is specialized for verbal representations, and the right for other modalities (Patterson et al., 2007).

COMMON MEMORY PROBLEMS AFTER BRAIN INJURY

Clients with brain injury can describe a wide variety of experiences that can indicate that their memory has been affected. These include:

"I know what I mean to do, but I don't remember to do it!" This sort of comment is really common after brain injury. It describes a "prospective" memory problem, or difficulty in retrieving intentions at the time we intended to act on them.

---

*All handouts are at the end of the chapter.

"I remember everything from decades ago, but I can't remember what I did yesterday!" People can be perplexed or frustrated that seemingly "useless" memories are still available, whereas newer memories are not, but actually this phenomenon is very common. Older memories are stored differently from newly formed memories, and the brain areas involved in the formation of new memories (i.e., encoding and consolidation processes) are particularly vulnerable to damage in common neurological conditions, including brain injury.

"I know that we went on a holiday a few weeks ago, but I don't have any memory of it, and I can't even remember where we went without checking my diary." This is a quotation from a client with damage to the hippocampus, who had severe difficulty forming new memories. This type of impairment can have important secondary effects on social and emotional functioning.

"I just can't remember things as well as I used to. I need to write things down so I can check them later; I can never seem to remember the names of new people I meet; and it's much harder to keep up at work nowadays." This type of comment is quite typical of people who still have a reasonable degree of episodic memory functioning, but have experienced a significant reduction from their preinjury level. Understanding the links between different cognitive systems (e.g., between attention and memory), and between different types of memory, can help people to identify their own strengths and weaknesses—and to adapt accordingly.

MAKING THE LINKS

Probably the biggest factor to influence memory is attention. Without attention, a person cannot have explicit memory, so the strategies described in Chapter 3 of this book can also be useful for memory. Moreover, the factors that influence attention, such as fatigue, exert a subsequent influence on memory, so clients and therapists need to be aware of these too.

Poor sleep can also have a negative impact on memory. We know that sleep is important in consolidating memories (Stickgold, 2005), so if sleep is disrupted, clients may remember things from the previous day less well than if they have had a good night's sleep. It is important to have a good sleep routine (going to bed and getting up at similar times every night), avoid caffeine after late afternoon, keep the bedroom dark and cool, and so forth. This is especially important if clients are needing to take on a lot of new information—for example, as part of taking a course or learning a new skill. Malley (Chapter 7, this volume) offers advice on managing fatigue.

We also know that mood can have a negative influence on memory. If clients are feeling anxious and/or low in mood, and especially if they have a lot of worries or tend to ruminate about the things that are now difficult in life, this can consume attentional capacity, leaving fewer resources (Watkins & Brown, 2002). Low mood can also result in biased thinking, so clients are more likely to recall negative memories when feeling low, and find it harder to access more positive memories (Matthews & Bradle, 1983; Eich, 1995). The mood management strategies described by Ford (Chapter 8, this volume) will be helpful here.

Some medications can also have an impact on memory, and on attention with subsequent effects on memory. Powell (2013) provides a useful review of this area. If clients have queries about the effects of the medications they are taking, it is best to ask the medical professionals involved in their care.

Finally, aging has a specific impact on memory, over and above the general effects of age on cognition (Rabbitt & Lowe, 2000). The strategies in the rest of this chapter can be useful for age-related changes in memory, as well as brain-injury-related changes.

ASSESSING MEMORY

The formal way to assess memory is to have a neuropsychological assessment conducted by (or under the supervision of) a qualified clinician. This can examine any likely changes in a client's memory ability, in addition to identifying memory strengths and challenges, and provide pointers toward strategies that might be particularly useful. If a neuropsychological assessment is feasible, it can be useful to identify answers to the following questions:

- Is the client's overall memory functioning in line with his or her intellectual ability, or has there been a likely reduction?

- If there is a relative impairment, at what level is the client currently functioning?

- Are there any differences in memory for visual versus verbal material? If so, can one type of memory be used to compensate for the other?

- Is there a difference in the client's ability to recall versus recognize information? Recognition is usually "easier" than recall, as there is an inherent cue. However, if there is a relative benefit for recognition over recall (e.g., if the person is within the lower 5% of the population for recall but at the population average for recognition), this may mean that the memory difficulties have a more frontal or executive basis than a purely mnemonic one. This often means that a client will benefit from the provision of cues and careful structuring of information.

- How is the client's ability to remember information after a delay? If there is a disproportionate loss of information after a short delay, this implies that memory strategies and external aids need to be used quickly, before the memory trace has had the opportunity to decay.

- Are there any other observations that suggest particular strategies might be useful? For example, if a list-learning task is used, is there evidence of semantic clustering or other forms of spontaneous strategy use? It is also informative to examine the cognitive profile more broadly: Is there likely to be an impact of attentional problems on memory? Does the client have strengths in planning and organization, which might indicate that external memory aids would be a good method of compensation for memory difficulties?

Memory questionnaires completed by clients and/or other persons who know the clients well can provide information on the functional impact of the clients' memory difficulties. Comparing self- and informant-rated versions of a questionnaire can also shed light on a client's insight into his or her memory difficulties (though note that this comparison relies upon the informant's accurate reporting). Handout 4.2 offers one such example.

It can also be useful to keep a checklist of frequent memory mistakes; see Handout 4.3 (adapted from a diary created by Alan Sunderland; Sunderland, Harris, & Baddeley, 1984). This can also be used as a way of monitoring the success of memory strategies.

REHABILITATION: THE EVIDENCE

The sections below on strategies and behavioral experiments are influenced by cognitive psychology experiments that have identified factors or conditions associated with improved memory performance. Here are two well-known examples:

1. In studies informing the "levels-of-processing" hypothesis formulated by Fergus Craik and colleagues (see, e.g., Craik & Lockhart, 1972), information that has been encoded "deeply" is better remembered than information that has been encoded in a "shallow" manner. For example, in a word-learning task, thinking about a word's meaning will result in better retrieval than thinking about how a word sounds. This finding is linked to the specific strategies of making associations, mnemonics, and PQRST, but it is also a general principle to follow in any learning situation.

2. We know that there are context effects in memory, thanks to an inventive study by Godden and Baddeley (1975) in which members of a student diving club were given information to learn while they were either in the water or at the side of the water on dry land, and were then tested on this information in the same pair of settings. Memory was better if the retrieval situation matched the encoding situation than if there was a mismatch between the encoding and retrieval conditions. A similar finding has been obtained more recently in a medical education setting: If student doctors learn about anatomy when they are wearing scrubs, they recall better when wearing scrubs, but if they learn in their own clothes, they remember better in their own clothes (Finn, Patten, & McLachlan, 2010). This type of finding is linked to strategies such as mental retracing (described later in this chapter).

Other strategies are based on studies more specifically about rehabilitation—for example, a series of studies on "errorless learning" conducted by Barbara A. Wilson and colleagues (see Wilson, 1999). As a result of this work, we know that if people with memory impairment are taught new information in ways that minimize the number of errors they make, the eventual memory for the correct information is much better than when errors are made and corrected during the learning phase.

There has also been a lot of interest in the scientific literature and popular press about "brain training," particularly for improving working memory. It is beyond the scope of this book to review the literature on brain training, and much of this research has focused either on children with developmental disorders or on healthy older adults, rather than on people with brain injury. However, at present, the general consensus from neuroscientists in the field of rehabilitation is that repetitive practice on computerized cognitive tasks improves performance on those tasks. These improvements do not necessarily transfer to everyday life, and they do not necessarily improve the underlying cognitive ability (i.e., participants in brain training studies get better on the tasks used in training, and sometimes on tests that are similar to those used in training, but improvements in day-to-day functioning are seldom observed).

The international group of clinicians and researchers known as INCOG (mentioned in Chapter 3) recently supported these conclusions, stating that "there is good evidence for the integration of internal and external compensatory memory strategies that are implemented using instructional procedures . . . the evidence for the efficacy of restorative strategies currently remains weak" (Velíkonja et al., 2014, p. 369).

EXPLORING MEMORY AND ITS PROBLEMS WITH CLIENTS

What Is Memory?

Before introducing the activities and strategies described below, you will probably find it helpful to do some basic psychoeducation with clients, looking at different memory types and processes, the ways the brain works in relation to these different types/processes, and some common difficulties. This can help them to start considering their own memory strengths and challenges. Handout 4.4 offers an accessible explanation of the different types of memory.

Playing what we at The Oliver Zangwill Centre call "Kim's game" can provide a really helpful starting point to help clients realize that they already have some resources that will be helpful in managing the memory difficulty. Prepare a tray with 10–12 different items (see Figure 10.3 in Prince, Chapter 10, this volume, for a picture of such a tray). Name and show each item to clients for 2 minutes; then cover the items up, and ask clients to write down as many items as they can remember. Once the clients have finished, ask them how they tried to memorize the items. Are any strategies already being used? Remember, the intent of this activity is to help clients understand whether they are already using strategies, rather than to focus on how many items they remember.

What Can Happen to Memory after Brain Injury?

Handout 4.5 outlines some common problems with memory, supported by real-life examples. Discuss these with clients, and ask which of the problems they have or might have experienced themselves.

Completing a Memory Diary

Ask each client to complete a 7-day memory diary (see the example in Handout 4.3). Then review the diary together, to identify whether any particular memory slips happen more often than others. Filling in this diary is in itself a memory task, so it can be helpful to set up a supporting system collaboratively with the client. This might involve identifying a particular time of day when using the diary is likely to be convenient, setting an alarm on a mobile phone to remind the person to complete the diary, and/or asking the client to complete the diary along with a family member.

REHABILITATION STRATEGIES

Don't be surprised if, as you read this section, you will find that you know some of these strategies already and may even be using a few with clients; we're just putting names to them.

There are two main types of memory strategies: "internal" and "external" strategies. Some strategies include elements of both types, however, and it can be really good to combine strategies involving each type.

1. Internal strategies are new ways of taking in information to make it more memorable and/or easier for us to retrieve, such as imagining turning a story into a picture to help us remember it. This is "making the best use of the memory we have."
2. External strategies involve using devices to contain the information to be remembered, or to remind us to complete particular tasks. An example is to write a shopping list, or to set a phone alarm as a reminder to send a birthday card. This type of method means that we don't have to rely on memory so much, but we do still need to remember to use the strategies.

The following principles form the basis for all memory strategies:

* Identify the information to be remembered.
* Minimize the amount of information to be remembered.
* Structure the information to learn, and make this structure as meaningful as possible.
* Define a cue for retrieving the information.
* Rehearse what needs to be remembered.

The important thing about any strategy is that it needs to be personal to the client. We are all much more likely to remember something if we have generated and encoded the information so that it is meaningful for us. For example, below are strategies clients have thought of for themselves that therapists probably wouldn't have come up with:

* 49 (relating to a reference number)—the last lottery number.
* 27 (relating to a house number)—3 × 9.
* Sharon—the same name as my sister.

Some clients find it helpful to use multimodal or bizarre connections to support memory. However, note that this can be challenging for those who tend toward concrete thinking or for people with very severe memory problems.

Sometimes clients dislike the idea of using strategies, and of course this makes it less likely that such clients will engage with the process of trialling and adopting strategies. When this comes to light, you will need to identify *why* a particular client is opposed to the idea. Does he or she think that using strategies is "lazy"? That it will make his or her memory worse? That it will make them look "different" or incapable? Or something else entirely? Taking time to explore such beliefs is important, as it validates the client's position, builds the therapeutic alliance, and allows for the collaborative planning of experiments to test the beliefs. Useful activities (to give just a few examples) can include listing the pros and cons of using and of *not* using strategies; conducting Internet searches to investigate the effects of memory aid use on memory ability; and conducting surveys of memory aids used by people with and without brain injury, and/or surveys of people's perceptions about memory aid use by others.

Instructional Methods to Support Memory

Errorless Learning

As noted earlier in this chapter, when people with memory impairment learn new information, they do better if they avoid making mistakes during learning. One reason for this is that making mistakes can be confusing; another reason is that errorless learning can make the learning process more enjoyable than a procedure that incorporates errors. So if clients are unsure of something, encourage them to check the information, rather than to guess incorrectly and risk getting a mistake "stuck" in memory!

As a therapist, you can often help a client learn or relearn skills by means of errorless learning. You can do this through collaboration with the client on developing a checklist for a task, written in the client's own words—for example, learning a new recipe, or finding the way from one location to another.

Also, *go slowly!* Mistakes crop up more easily if clients are rushing. It can help a client to have detailed instructions for a new task, and/or someone to guide the client through this process.

Spaced Retrieval

It's good not only to repeat the information that clients are trying to learn, but to do so over increasing time intervals (e.g., right away, then after a 1-minute delay, and then at 2-minute, 5-minute, and 30-minute intervals) and in a varying format (e.g., changing the order of what's to be recalled, or saying it aloud and then writing it down).

Retrieval Practice and the Overlearning Principle

Studies show that the more often people successfully retrieve information, the stronger their memory for it gets. This phenomenon is known as "retrieval practice" (Roediger & Butler, 2011). Encourage clients to keep practicing and testing themselves; as the old adage goes, practice makes perfect! Emphasize the overlearning principle (i.e., that repeated practice at a task embeds it in our memories, so rather than having to think about it a great deal, it becomes virtually automatic).

Combined Approaches to Learning New Information

These instructional methods can (and should) be combined, so that practice takes place over increasing intervals, with lots of testing, and with the chances of errors eliminated or kept to an absolute minimum. Find real-life, meaningful examples for clients to practice with; for instance, ask clients to learn the phone number of a person or service they call often. Alternatively, think of other information it would be helpful for clients to memorize (e.g., relatives' birthdays, computer passwords, addresses).

Internal Strategies

Making Associations

Memory can be supported by linking things to be learned with other things that are meaningful or personal to a client. Here are some examples:

* Associating a new activity with an existing routine (e.g., checking a to-do list at break times, taking medication at mealtimes).
* Learning a new name by making a link (e.g., "Carol with the curly hair").
* Leaving a pair of walking shoes or boots by the door, to remind a client that he or she is meeting a friend for a walk.

Handout 4.6 explains this strategy and offers some opportunities to practice making associations. Support clients in reflecting on how well the associations worked.

Chunking

"Chunking" is a method of splitting information into smaller or otherwise more manageable groups or units, and thus making it easier to store. Chunking information into smaller groups is particularly useful for numbers (e.g., 462 537 981 is easier to remember than 462537981). Another example of chunking is grouping information together into meaningful units or categories (e.g., by first letter, type of product, or type of task); this can be helpful for remembering items on a shopping list or a to-do list). Handout 4.7 explains the strategy and offers some practice.

Keywords

Using "keywords" can be a good way of breaking down a large amount of information so that it is easier to remember. This takes up less room in the memory system and can be enough to cue the remaining information. For example, remembering "I need to buy ingredients to make lasagna" is easier than remembering "I need to buy ground beef, tomato sauce, milk, parmesan, and pasta sheets."

Visual Imagery

Making a mental picture of something can help support memory. This can be an especially important strategy if clients have problems with verbal memory. Handout 4.8 offers some examples and practice suggestions.

Mental Blackboard

The "mental blackboard" is a visualization strategy in which clients imagine carrying a blackboard or notepad around inside their head. Encourage them to visualize actually writing/drawing things they need to remember on the blackboard. Checking their mental blackboard throughout the day will help them to keep on track, though it is important not to put too much or too little information on the blackboard. Handout 4.9 shows some examples. The mental blackboard strategy can be used in combination with the attention beam strategy described in Chapter 3: Encourage clients to use external alarms or catchphrases (e.g., "Am I on track?" or "Stop and think!") to prompt themselves to turn their attention beam inward toward the mental blackboard at regular intervals.

Memory Palace

The "memory palace" technique is a combination of using associations and visualization in a place that is very familiar to a client and thus can easily be recalled to memory. The client imagines a clear route through the "palace" and identifies distinctive features. Things that need to be remembered are associated with these features, and can be recalled as the client follows the imaginary route. Handout 4.10 explains the strategy to clients and offers an example and practice activity.

Mental Retracing

"Mental retracing" is an effective way for clients to review their movements, actions, and thoughts from an earlier point in time to facilitate recall of a piece of information. Here is an example:

> "Where are my keys? They're not on the key holder. I remember locking the car—then I came into the house. Jamie asked what we were having for dinner. I noticed the mail on the table and went straight over to it, as there was a letter I was expecting. I remember opening the letter—I'll check if the keys are on the table."

Ask clients to use mental retracing to recall when they last made a phone call, what they had for dinner on Saturday, when they last took a taxi, and what was the last thing they spent money on.

Mnemonics

"Mnemonics" are usually devices to support memory, and can be good for remembering rules, lists of things, or a sequence of words. They can take the form of rhymes (e.g., "I before E except after C") or can use the first letters of words (e.g., "Richard Of York Gave Battle In Vain" to remember the colors of the rainbow). Clients can also make up stories to help them remember. Encourage clients to think of mnemonics they know already. Handout 4.11 explains the strategies, gives examples, and provides suggestions for practice.

Encourage clients to think of examples to use in real-life situations for things they have to remember.

The PQRST Strategy

"PQRST" is a strategy that clients can use when studying or reading to assist them to take in and remember what the information is about (see Handout 4.12). Though we have classed it as an internal strategy, it can be considered an external strategy if it is done in a written format and referred to by the client later on. The letters stand for the following:

P = Preview: Clients skim or look over a piece of writing to get an idea of what it is generally about.

Q = Question: The next step is for clients to think about what questions they are hoping to answer by reading the information (who/what/where/when/why/how?).

R = Read: Clients then read the piece of writing slowly to take in what it is about.

S = Summarize: After reading, clients sum up the essence of the piece in their own words.

T = Test: Finally, clients check that they have answered all the questions they originally wanted to answer.

Select some newspaper or magazine articles and think up a set of questions about them. Ask the client to read one, then ask the client the questions. Then try the same thing with another story using PQRST. See how much they take in and with each, encourage reflection on why this might be.

Mindmaps

"Mindmaps" are visual representations of thoughts or concepts. Mindmaps are particularly useful for studying or learning new information about a topic, as they incorporate a number of the internal strategies previously outlined; but as they are put down on paper, they also function as external memory aids. For example, some clients find mindmaps useful aids in preparing for meetings or presentations, as they chunk and link key points together in a visual way, which can be easier for the clients to follow.

External Strategies

As the name indicates, external strategies are the strategies that we can see! There are lots to choose from, with the most popular ones including smartphones, whiteboards, wall calendars, Filofaxes or other types of personal organizers/planners, and notebooks.

When you are helping clients to use external memory aids, it is important to work collaboratively to identify which types of aids are likely to fit with their lifestyles and values. A good starting point is to consider how they remembered various types of information in the past, how they remember these things now, and whether the method or methods they are using now are effective (see Handout 4.2). Some clients report feeling that memory aids will constrain them and mean that they are unable to live spontaneously. Others feel that using aids is somehow "cheating" by not testing their memories, or may worry that memory aids will make them look "different" or exaggerate their problems. It is important to explore the meaning of using a memory aid with each client before proceeding, as having this understanding helps both you and the client to develop a more acceptable and effective memory system. Use the information clients have gathered while exploring their cognitive profile to help them identify areas that could be supported by use of a memory aid (e.g., a calendar or notebook for appointments, names, and addresses; a to-do list, a mood log). Use the Goal Management Framework (GMF; see Winegardner, Chapter 5, this volume) to explore the pros and cons of each option, and to help the client reach a decision about which is best to use.

Once the choice has been made, it can be helpful to agree with the client on a protocol for using the aid (see the example in Handout 4.13). Clients may require a good deal of scaffolding to help them build the habit of using a memory aid. Structured regimens can be set up either at home or in a rehabilitation center, with support from family or staff members. Morning diary-planning sessions can review what is on the agenda for the day. This can be followed by a lunchtime catch-up to review whether clients are on track for achieving the day's goals, and a session at the end of the day to check that everything has been done and to look ahead to the following day.

In the context of a rehabilitation center, clients are prompted to bring their memory aids to sessions, to check their aids as appropriate, and to note down appointments and to-do list items in the moment. Direct prompts to use an aid can be given at first, but such prompts should be gradually "faded" to indirect prompts, with the goal of eventual independence as the habit develops. Weekly goals can be set around the use of memory aids—ideally, to support valued occupational participation—and frequency of use and level of independence can be monitored to track progress.

In the community, it is likely that as a therapist you will need to enlist the help of caregivers, family members, friends, or colleagues to support building a routine, with an emphasis on consistency and repetition. Some families find it helpful to have a weekly planning meeting, at which diaries and calendars can be coordinated for the week ahead. This can also serve to normalize the use of memory aids in everyday life.

Smartphones and Other Electronic Devices

How things have changed in the last few years! Many people are starting to use electronic devices, particularly mobile phones, to support memory. Not only can we automatically save contacts, access a calendar, create to-do lists, and use the camera function of a smartphone to capture images to cue memory, but we have access to apps that can perform a wealth of other functions. In fact, think of what you'd like an app for, and it's probably out there! Apps can be used successfully for budgeting and keeping track of money, managing to-do lists, and task reminders. Needless to say, new apps are being developed all the time. The U.K. National Health Service has developed a Health Apps Library (*http://apps.nhs.uk*), which serves as a useful guide to apps that have been reviewed by clinicians to ensure that they are relevant, accurate, and secure.

The great advantages of mobile devices are that they are easily portable, and that the majority of us are used to having our phones with us most of the time. Clients may, however, need support to use the necessary smartphone functions and apps, and the strategies outlined previously can be used to provide such support. Psychologists in Toronto have recently been evaluating programs for helping memory-impaired people to learn to use smart phones, with good results (Svoboda, Richards, Leach, & Mertens, 2012). If clients are not confident or able to set reminders on their phones, then you may need to collaborate, so that a relative, friend, or caregiver programs an agreed-upon set of reminders into the client's phone, with regular reviews to monitor usefulness and update reminder schedules. Alternatively, clients can use an externally managed reminder system such as NeuroPage, which sends reminder text messages to clients' mobile phones or pagers according to a previously specified schedule. These messages can be reminders of routine tasks (e.g., "At 10:00 A.M., take your blood pressure medication"), or general messages to support use of other strategies (e.g., twice per day, "Have you checked your to-do list?"). The results of several research trials have demonstrated that NeuroPage and other similar systems are effective in helping people to remember and achieve day-to-day goals (e.g., Wilson, Emslie, Quirk, & Evans, 2001).

Of course, it is all too easy to lose a mobile phone. Synchronizing data frequently with another device can minimize frustration should this occur, but remember that it is important for clients to get into the routine of doing this, whether on a daily or a weekly basis. Various apps such as "Find My iPhone" and "If Found Lock Screen" can also be helpful in tracking the location of a phone, and providing good samaritans with the necessary information to return a lost phone to its owner.

Memory Notebooks and Personal Organizers

Memory notebooks and personal organizers can be used in much the same way as their electronic counterparts, and it is important to note that some clients prefer pencil and paper to technology. Most contain address books, calendars, notepads, to-do lists, and so on. However, they do *not* remind a client to use them! The neuropsychologist Narinder Kapur recommends using a simple electronic reminding device, such as a text message or vibrating watch alert, to encourage the use of paper diaries (Kapur, Glisky, & Wilson, 2004).

COMPLETING A MEMORY PROFILE

Clients may wish to complete a copy of the memory profile sheet (see Handout 4.14) to add to their portfolios. Support clients in using their knowledge of their injury, their day-to-day experiences, and the information in this chapter to identify:

- The things they need to remember.
- What strategies they are currently using, which ones work, and which ones need more modification/testing.
- Their memory strengths and challenges (e.g., verbal vs. visual memory).
- Whether there are any new strategies they would like to try, and, if so, how these would fit into their lives and routines.

Work with the clients to put this information into their memory and planning systems in the ways that have most meaning to them, and encourage them to conduct trials of these methods. Often a client likes to have a visual representation of his or her personal memory system (see Handout 4.15).

BRINGING IT ALL TOGETHER

As with anything new, clients will need to practice using their memory systems consistently. Suggest that they try a strategy for a month, monitor how it's working, and then review it. One difficulty that clients sometimes experience is that, due to reduced occupational and social participation, there isn't actually very much to put into a memory system, and this can be very demotivating. "What's the point in checking my daily planner when there's hardly anything in it?" In this instance, some creativity may be required. If clients are working on a project as part of their rehabilitation, explore how the memory system can be used to support completion of project-related tasks. Perhaps a client has a social participation goal that involves contacting friends to make arrangements to meet. For this client, memory aids can support remembering to make phone calls; planning a venue, route, and transportation; thinking of topics of conversation for the meeting; and recalling what was said for next time. If the client is working on domestic roles, reminders can be set for doing daily or weekly tasks, making shopping lists, and the like. Alternatively, you could assign some homework that relies on doing something on a particular day. You could ask the client to phone you the day before his or her next appointment to confirm the appointment, or ask the client to drop something off at the reception desk when he or she leaves your session. Collaborate with the client, family, friends, and other professionals to ensure that the client uses the memory system to support every aspect of daily life. Even something as simple as planning which TV programs to watch during the week can serve as a way of embedding the system's use.

CASE STUDY

Because attention and memory are so closely linked, the case study in Chapter 3 on attention also covers the memory work completed with Jeff.

REFERENCES

Baddeley, A. D., & Hitch, G. J. (1974). Working memory. *Psychology of Learning and Motivation, 8,* 47–89.

Craik, F. I., & Lockhart, R. S. (1972). Levels of processing: A framework for memory research. *Journal of Verbal Learning and Verbal Behavior, 11*(6), 671–684.

Eich, E. (1995). Searching for mood dependent memory. *Psychological Science, 6*(2), 67–75.

Finn, G. M., Patten, D., & McLachlan, J. C. (2010). The impact of wearing scrubs on contextual learning. *Medical Teacher, 32*(5), 381–384.

Fish, J., Wilson, B. A., & Manly, T. (2010). The assessment and rehabilitation of prospective memory problems in people with neurological disorders: A review. *Neuropsychological Rehabilitation, 20*(2), 161–179.

Fletcher, P. C., & Henson, R. N. A. (2001). Frontal lobes and human memory. *Brain, 124*(5), 849–881.

Godden, D. R., & Baddeley, A. D. (1975). Context-dependent memory in two natural environments: On land and underwater. *British Journal of Psychology, 66,* 325–331.

Kapur, N., Glisky, E. L., & Wilson, B. A. (2004). Technological memory aids for people with memory deficits. *Neuropsychological Rehabilitation, 14*(1–2), 41–60.

Kelley, W. M., Miezin, F. M., McDermott, K. B., Buckner, R. L., Raichle, M. E., Cohen, N. J., . . . Petersen, S. E. (1998). Hemispheric specialization in human dorsal frontal cortex and medial temporal lobe for verbal and nonverbal memory encoding. *Neuron, 20*(5), 927–936.

Mathews, A., & Bradle, B. (1983). Mood and the self-reference bias in recall. *Behaviour Research and Therapy, 21*(3), 233–239.

Patterson, K., Nestor, P. J., & Rogers, T. T. (2007). Where do you know what you know?: The representation of semantic knowledge in the human brain. *Nature Reviews Neuroscience, 8*(12), 976–987.

Powell, J. E. (2013). The effects of prescribed and recreational drug use on cognitive functioning. In L. H. Goldstein & J. E. McNeil (Eds.), *Clinical neuropsychology: A practical guide to assessment and management for clinicians* (2nd ed., pp. 105–128). Chichester, UK: Wiley-Blackwell.

Rabbitt, P., & Lowe, C. (2000). Patterns of cognitive ageing. *Psychological Research, 63*(3–4), 308–316.

Roediger, H. L., & Butler, A. C. (2011). The critical role of retrieval practice in long-term retention. *Trends in Cognitive Sciences, 15*(1), 20–27.

Squire, L. R., & Knowlton, B. J. (1995). Memory, hippocampus, and brain systems. In M. S. Gazzaniga (Ed.), *The cognitive neurosciences* (pp. 825–837). Cambridge, MA: MIT Press.

Squire, L. R., & Zola-Morgan, S. (1991). The medial temporal lobe memory system. *Science, 253*(5026), 1380–1386.

Stickgold, R. (2005). Sleep-dependent memory consolidation. *Nature, 437*(7063), 1272–1278.

Sunderland, A., Harris, J. E., & Baddeley, A. D. (1984). Assessing everyday memory after severe head injury. In J. E. Harris & P. E. Morris (Eds.), *Everyday memory, actions and absent-mindedness* (pp. 191–206). London: Academic Press.

Svoboda, E., Richards, B., Leach, L., & Mertens, V. (2012). PDA and smartphone use by individuals with moderate-to-severe memory impairment: Application of a theory-driven training programme. *Neuropsychological Rehabilitation, 22*(3), 408–427.

Tulving, E. (2002). Episodic memory: From mind to brain. *Annual Review of Psychology, 53*(1), 1–25.

Velikonja, D., Tate, R., Ponsford, J., McIntyre, A., Janzen, S., & Bayley, M. (2014). INCOG recommendations for management of cognition following traumatic brain injury: Part V. Memory. *Journal of Head Trauma Rehabilitation, 29*(4), 369–386.

Watkins, E., & Brown, R. G. (2002). Rumination and executive function in depression: An experimental study. *Journal of Neurology, Neurosurgery and Psychiatry, 72*(3), 400–402.

Wilson, B. A. (1999). *Case studies in neuropsychological rehabilitation.* New York: Oxford University Press.

FURTHER READING

Evans, J. J. (2013). Disorders of memory. In L. H. Goldstein & J. E. McNeil (Eds.), *Clinical neuro-psychology: A practical guide to assessment and management for clinicians* (2nd ed., pp. 159–194). Chichester, UK: Wiley-Blackwell.

Max Planck Institute for Human Development and Stanford Center on Longevity. (2014, October 15). *A consensus on the brain training industry from the scientific community.* Retrieved from *http://longevity3.stanford.edu/blog/2014/10/15/the-consensus-on-the-brain-training-industry-from-the-scientific-community*

Ptak, R., der Linden, M. V., & Schnider, A. (2010). Cognitive rehabilitation of episodic memory disorders: From theory to practice. *Frontiers in Human Neuroscience, 4,* 57.

Wilson, B. A. (1987). *Rehabilitation of memory.* New York: Guilford Press.

Wilson, B. A., Emslie, H. C., Quirk, K., & Evans, J. J. (2001). Reducing everyday memory and planning problems by means of a paging system: A randomized control crossover study. *Journal of Neurology, Neurosurgery, and Psychiatry, 70*(4), 477–482.

Brain Areas Involved in Memory

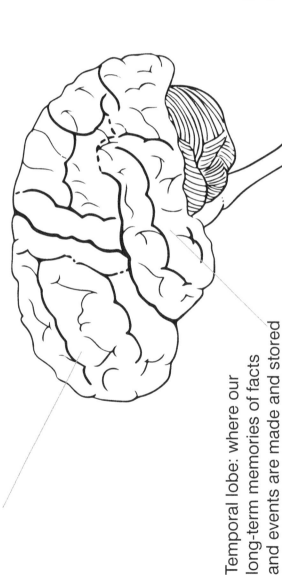

Frontal lobe: involved in "working" memory and accessing information from long-term memory

Temporal lobe: where our long-term memories of facts and events are made and stored

Hippocampus: involved in new learning

From *The Brain Injury Rehabilitation Workbook*, edited by Rachel Winson, Barbara A. Wilson, and Andrew Bateman. Copyright © 2017 The Guilford Press. Permission to photocopy this handout is granted to purchasers of this book for personal use or for use with individual clients (see copyright page for details). Purchasers can download additional copies of this handout (see the box at the end of the table of contents).

How Do I Remember Things?

Complete this form, indicating how you currently remember to do the following activities ("What do you use now?"), whether you have any problems remembering, and whether there is anything else you think you could use instead.

Activity	What do you use now?	Do you have any problems remembering to do this?	Is there anything else you could use instead?
Birthdays			
Appointments			
Weekly activities (such as putting out the trash)			
Buying items when shopping			
Keeping track of money you've spent			
Paying bills			
Telephoning friends and family			

(continued)

From *The Brain Injury Rehabilitation Workbook*, edited by Rachel Winson, Barbara A. Wilson, and Andrew Bateman. Copyright © 2017 The Guilford Press. Permission to photocopy this handout is granted to purchasers of this book for personal use or for use with individual clients (see copyright page for details). Purchasers can download additional copies of this handout (see the box at the end of the table of contents).

Activity	What do you use now?	Do you have any problems remembering to do this?	Is there anything else you could use instead?
Answering letters			
Things you need to do at some point in future (such as redecorate a room)			
Things you need to do today (such as get meat out of the freezer)			
Taking messages on the telephone			
Names of people you meet			
How to get to new places			
Where you've been and what you've been doing			
Conversations you've had with people			
Social arrangements			
Where you've put something			

Memory Diary

Every evening for 1 week, go through the diary with _____ (fill in the person's name here) and indicate how many times each thing happened to you during that day. If you forget to fill it in one evening, don't guess—just leave that day blank.

	Day						
	1	2	3	4	5	6	7
1. Forgetting where you have put something. Losing things around the house.							
2. Failing to recognize a place that you are told you have often been to before.							
3. Finding a television story difficult to follow.							
4. Not remembering a change in your daily routine, such as a change in the place where something is kept, or a change in the time something happens. Following your old routine by mistake.							
5. Having to go back to check whether you have done something that you meant to do.							
6. When thinking of the past, forgetting when something happened—for example, whether it was yesterday or last week.							
7. Completely forgetting to take things with you, or leaving things behind and having to go back and fetch them.							
8. Forgetting that you were told something yesterday or a few days ago, and having to be reminded of it.							
9. Starting to read something (a book or an article in a newspaper or magazine) without realizing you have already read it.							

(continued)

From *The Brain Injury Rehabilitation Workbook*, edited by Rachel Winson, Barbara A. Wilson, and Andrew Bateman. Copyright © 2017 The Guilford Press. Permission to photocopy this handout is granted to purchasers of this book for personal use or for use with individual clients (see copyright page for details). Purchasers can download additional copies of this handout (see the box at the end of the table of contents).

Memory Diary *(page 2 of 3)*

	Day						
	1	2	3	4	5	6	7
10. Letting yourself speak for too long about unimportant or irrelevant things.							
11. Failing to recognize, by sight, close relatives or friends that you meet frequently.							
12. Having difficulty in picking up a new skill—for example, having difficulty in learning a new game or in working some new gadget after you have practiced once or twice.							
13. Finding that a word is "on the tip of your tongue": You know what it is, but you can't find it.							
14. Completely forgetting to do things you said you would do, and things you planned to do.							
15. Forgetting important details of what you did or what happened to you the day before.							
16. When talking to someone, forgetting what you have just said. Maybe saying, "What was I talking about?"							
17. When reading a newspaper or magazine, being unable to follow the thread of a story, or losing track of what it is about.							
18. Forgetting to tell somebody something important. Perhaps forgetting to pass on a message or remind someone of something.							
19. Forgetting important details about yourself (e.g., your birth date, or where you live).							
20. Getting the details of what someone has told you mixed up or confused.							
21. Telling someone a story or joke that you have told the person once already.							

(continued)

	Day						
	1	2	3	4	5	6	7
22. Forgetting details of things you do regularly. Details of what to do, or at what time to do it.							
23. Finding that the faces of famous people, when you see them on television or in photographs, look unfamiliar.							
24. Forgetting where things are normally kept, or looking for them in the wrong place.							
25a. Getting lost or turning in the wrong direction on a journey, on a walk, or in a building, where you have *often* been before.							
25b. Getting lost or turning in the wrong direction on a journey, on a walk, or in a building, where you have been only *once or twice* before.							
26. Doing some routine thing twice by mistake—for example, putting two teabags in your cup instead of one, or going to brush/comb your hair when you have just done so.							
27. Repeating to someone what you have just told them, or asking them the same question twice.							
28. Having to be nagged before you do something.							
29. Missing a TV program you wanted to watch.							
30. Remembering to do something, but not at the right time.							

Did you forget to do anything today? Did you have any other memory or concentration difficulties? If so, please describe: _____

Adapted from Sunderland, Harris, and Baddeley (1984). Used by permission of Elsevier Ltd.

What Is Memory?

Episodic memory: Memory for events

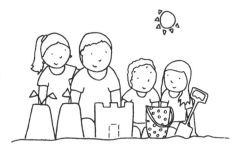

Prospective memory: Remembering to do things
in the future

Semantic memory: Memory for facts

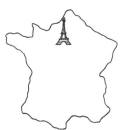

Working memory: Holding information in mind
and using it

Procedural memory: Memory for skills
and movements

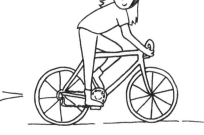

Priming: Perhaps not remembering having seen or heard
something before, but understanding it more quickly
the second time around

Conditioning: Associating one thing with another,
without being conscious of the link

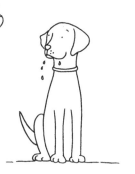

(continued)

From *The Brain Injury Rehabilitation Workbook*, edited by Rachel Winson, Barbara A. Wilson, and Andrew Bateman. Copyright © 2017 The Guilford Press. Permission to photocopy this handout is granted to purchasers of this book for personal use or for use with individual clients (see copyright page for details). Purchasers can download additional copies of this handout (see the box at the end of the table of contents).

There are three stages of memory:

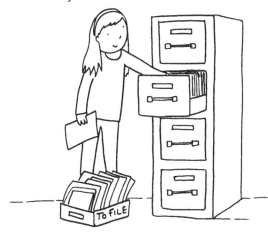

1. Encoding (taking it in)

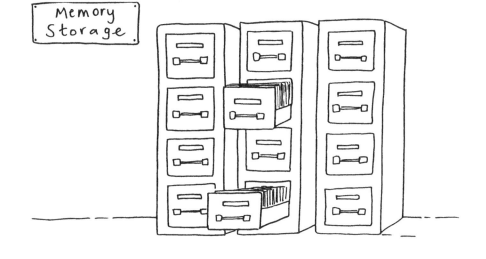

2. Storage (keeping it)

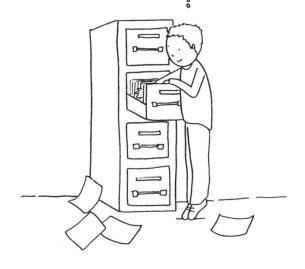

3. Retrieval (finding it again when you need it)

Do You Ever Have . . . ?

As we have learned, memory for visual information and memory for verbal information are supported by different parts of the brain. Because brain injuries are rarely neat and symmetrical, this means that many people will have more difficulty with one type of memory than another. Do you ever have . . .

- Difficulty remembering after a delay or distraction?

- Problems with learning new information?

- Better memory for events from long ago, and comparatively weaker memory for recent events ("I remember everything from decades ago, but I can't remember what I did yesterday!")?

- Difficulty remembering to do things ("I know what I mean to do, but I don't remember to do it!")?

- Trouble remembering events that have happened ("I know that we went on a vacation a few weeks ago, but I don't have any memory of it")?

- Problems with remembering names and faces ("I can never seem to remember the names of new people I meet")?

- Difficulty finding the right word ("It's on the tip of my tongue")?

From *The Brain Injury Rehabilitation Workbook*, edited by Rachel Winson, Barbara A. Wilson, and Andrew Bateman. Copyright © 2017 The Guilford Press. Permission to photocopy this handout is granted to purchasers of this book for personal use or for use with individual clients (see copyright page for details). Purchasers can download additional copies of this handout (see the box at the end of the table of contents).

Making the Links

Memory can be supported by linking things with something meaningful or personal to you. This strategy can help you:

- Remember to do a new activity (e.g., take medication at mealtimes).
- Learn new names (e.g., "Carol with the curly hair").
- Remember items on a list (e.g., dishwashing liquid, soap, shampoo—all have bubbles).
- Prompt you to do things (e.g., leave your walking shoes or boots by the door to remind you that you are meeting a friend for a walk).

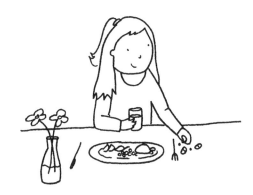

1. On a separate sheet of paper, write down the first thing you think of when you hear these words:

summer	seaside
telephone	glasses
football	keys
New York	London
computer	Tom Cruise

Now look at your associations. Can you remember the original words?

2. Now do some practical examples.

- How would you link a new activity to something that you already do?
- What associations could you use to remember the names of your therapists?
- How could you associate items on a shopping list to help you to remember them?
- What other items could you put in places to prompt you?

From *The Brain Injury Rehabilitation Workbook*, edited by Rachel Winson, Barbara A. Wilson, and Andrew Bateman. Copyright © 2017 The Guilford Press. Permission to photocopy this handout is granted to purchasers of this book for personal use or for use with individual clients (see copyright page for details). Purchasers can download additional copies of this handout (see the box at the end of the table of contents).

Chunking

Chunking is a way of splitting up a large amount of information into smaller groups that are easier to remember. It can be used with numbers, items on a list, or things you have to do.

1. How would you chunk these numbers to make them easier to remember?

   020 7946 0946   07700 900563   633500989

2. What about these items on a shopping list?

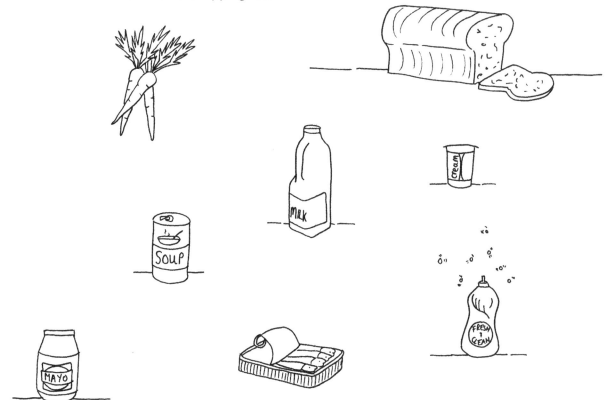

Carrots   Mayonnaise
Soup   Washing-up (dishwashing) liquid
Milk   Cream
Bread   Sardines

You could chunk these items by first letter:

B: Bread   C × 2: Carrots, cream
M × 2: Milk, mayonnaise   S × 2: Sardines, soup
W: Washing-up liquid

(continued)

From *The Brain Injury Rehabilitation Workbook*, edited by Rachel Winson, Barbara A. Wilson, and Andrew Bateman. Copyright © 2017 The Guilford Press. Permission to photocopy this handout is granted to purchasers of this book for personal use or for use with individual clients (see copyright page for details). Purchasers can download additional copies of this handout (see the box at the end of the table of contents).

Or you could chunk them by category:

    Dairy products: Cream, milk

    Lunch things: Soup, sardines, bread, mayonnaise, carrots

    Cleaning: Washing-up liquid

Could you chunk them in another way?

3. How can these tasks be chunked into categories?

Write letter to Janie	Vacuum floor	Phone Grandma
Send birthday card	Organize papers	Buy lightbulbs

The Mind's Eye

Making mental pictures can help you remember things:

- Names

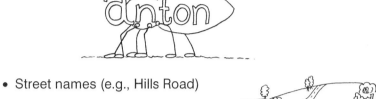

- Street names (e.g., Hills Road)

- Items on a list (e.g., cat food, teabags, toothpaste, soy sauce)

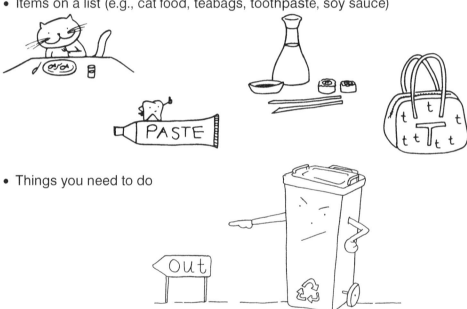

- Things you need to do

Make up your own mental images for these things:

1. Stephanie, Paul, Fred.
2. Oxford Street, Lincoln Road, Maple Grove.
3. On the way home, buy milk, three stamps from the post office, and eggs and flour for making a birthday cake.
4. Remember to record your favorite TV show and to feed the dog.

Draw on a separate sheet of paper one of the things on your to-do list for this week.

From *The Brain Injury Rehabilitation Workbook*, edited by Rachel Winson, Barbara A. Wilson, and Andrew Bateman. Copyright © 2017 The Guilford Press. Permission to photocopy this handout is granted to purchasers of this book for personal use or for use with individual clients (see copyright page for details). Purchasers can download additional copies of this handout (see the box at the end of the table of contents).

Mental Blackboard

Imagine that you have a blackboard in your mind. Visualize writing down or drawing pictures of the things you have to do. Don't put on too much or too little information.

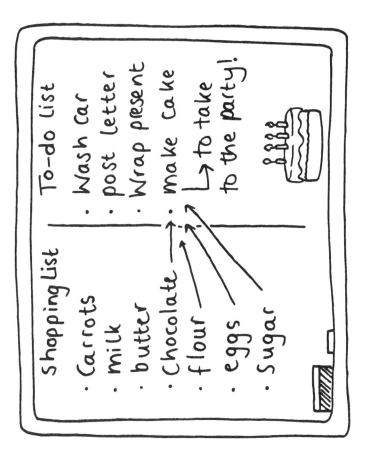

From *The Brain Injury Rehabilitation Workbook*, edited by Rachel Winson, Barbara A. Wilson, and Andrew Bateman. Copyright © 2017 The Guilford Press. Permission to photocopy this handout is granted to purchasers of this book for personal use or for use with individual clients (see copyright page for details). Purchasers can download additional copies of this handout (see the box at the end of the table of contents).

Memory Palace

Think of a familiar place you know really well. This is your "memory palace."
- List some distinctive features.
- Associate these features with items you need to remember.
- Imagine a clear route through your palace.
- "Walk through" the palace to recall the items.

For example, to remember you need to buy chicken, milk, toilet paper, carrots, and potatoes:
- Think of a familiar place, such as the large group room at the rehabilitation center.
- List some distinctive features: door, window, whiteboard, pool table with cues and balls.
- Make associations: door–chicken, window–milk, whiteboard–toilet paper, pool cues–carrots, pool balls–potatoes.
- Now make up a story: "There's a **chicken** making a lot of noise to get into the room (door), because it's raining **milk** outside (that's why the chicken is making so much noise). The chicken is looking at the person leading the group, who is writing on **toilet paper** (whiteboard). Someone has set up the pool table with **carrots** (pool cues) and **potatoes** (pool balls)."

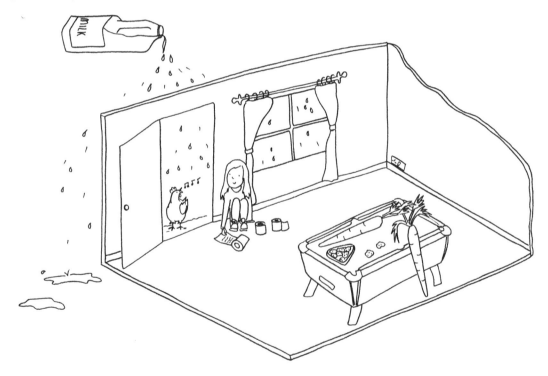

Create your own memory palace or mental walk to remember these items on a shopping list: eggs, butter, hot chocolate, soap, newspaper, batteries.

From *The Brain Injury Rehabilitation Workbook*, edited by Rachel Winson, Barbara A. Wilson, and Andrew Bateman. Copyright © 2017 The Guilford Press. Permission to photocopy this handout is granted to purchasers of this book for personal use or for use with individual clients (see copyright page for details). Purchasers can download additional copies of this handout (see the box at the end of the table of contents).

Mnemonics

Mnemonics are ways of learning information to make it easier to remember. Here are some examples.

Rhymes:

- "Thirty days hath September, April, June, and November . . ." to remember how many days each month has.
- "I before E except after C . . ." to remember spellings.

First-letter mnemonics:

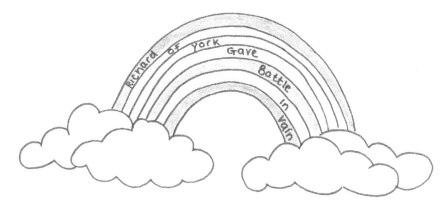

- "Richard Of York Gave Battle In Vain" to remember the colors of the rainbow: red, orange, yellow, green, blue, indigo, and violet.

Stories or phrases to remember words or numbers:

- A shopping list consisting of Shreddies, sugar, coffee, and toothpaste: "In the morning I get up and eat my Shreddies with sugar and have a cup of coffee. Then I brush my teeth."
- Personal identification numbers (PINs): "Do I climb frames?" = 2156 (number of letters in each word).
- Car license plate numbers: "Frances has 10 good-girl vehicles" = FH10 GGV.

Invent mnemonics for:

Your car license plate number, PIN, or some other important number.

A shopping list: furniture polish, teabags, milk, bananas.

From *The Brain Injury Rehabilitation Workbook*, edited by Rachel Winson, Barbara A. Wilson, and Andrew Bateman. Copyright © 2017 The Guilford Press. Permission to photocopy this handout is granted to purchasers of this book for personal use or for use with individual clients (see copyright page for details). Purchasers can download additional copies of this handout (see the box at the end of the table of contents).

The PQRST Strategy

PQRST is a strategy for reading or studying. Here's what the letters stand for:

P = **Preview**: Skim a piece of writing (read it very quickly) to get the gist of it.

Q = **Question:** Ask yourself what you want to find out from this piece of writing (who/what/where/when/why/how?).

R = **Read**: Read the piece slowly to take it in.

S = **Summarize:** Put the key facts in your own words.

T = **Test:** Check that you have found the information you wanted.

Now read an article in a newspaper/magazine or on a news app. Use PQRST as you read to remember the key facts. Then summarize the article to your therapist.

Give PQRST a try. You'll soon find that you automatically start thinking of questions to help you focus and remember when a news item has caught your eye.

From *The Brain Injury Rehabilitation Workbook*, edited by Rachel Winson, Barbara A. Wilson, and Andrew Bateman. Copyright © 2017 The Guilford Press. Permission to photocopy this handout is granted to purchasers of this book for personal use or for use with individual clients (see copyright page for details). Purchasers can download additional copies of this handout (see the box at the end of the table of contents).

Making Your Memory System Work

Morning Routine

- Check the day/date.
- Where are you? Do you need to go anywhere today? Do you need to take any morning medication?
- Check your diary: Have you got any appointments today? Do you need to set a reminder?
- Check your to-do list. Plan the best time to do each task. Set a reminder if you need to.

Midday

- Check your diary: Are you on track?

End-of-Day Review

- Review the day: Did you complete the tasks on your to-do list? If not, transfer them to your list for the next day.
- Look ahead to the next day: Do you have to go anywhere/do anything? Do you need to set reminders or prepare anything in advance?
- Do you need to take any evening medication?

Weekly Planning

- Meet with _____ (fill in name of person) to coordinate your diaries for the week ahead.
- Review the day (as usual).
- Look at the forthcoming week and make sure your diary matches _____'s. Look out for clashes or things that have been missed.
- Add any new appointments that have come through during the week.
- Make sure you're both clear about who is doing what over the next week.

From *The Brain Injury Rehabilitation Workbook*, edited by Rachel Winson, Barbara A. Wilson, and Andrew Bateman. Copyright © 2017 The Guilford Press. Permission to photocopy this handout is granted to purchasers of this book for personal use or for use with individual clients (see copyright page for details). Purchasers can download additional copies of this handout (see the box at the end of the table of contents).

My Memory Profile

What do I need to remember?	
Memory strengths	
Memory challenges	
Which strategies work?	
Which strategies don't work?	
My memory and planning system	
What next?	

From *The Brain Injury Rehabilitation Workbook*, edited by Rachel Winson, Barbara A. Wilson, and Andrew Bateman. Copyright © 2017 The Guilford Press. Permission to photocopy this handout is granted to purchasers of this book for personal use or for use with individual clients (see copyright page for details). Purchasers can download additional copies of this handout (see the box at the end of the table of contents).

My Memory System

EXTERNAL MEMORY SYSTEM

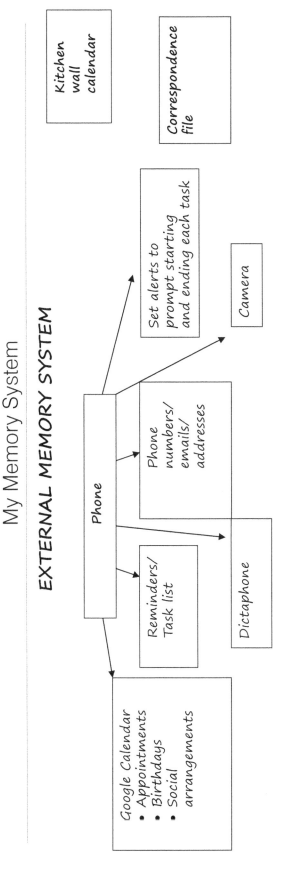

Kitchen wall calendar

Correspondence file

Phone

Set alerts to prompt starting and ending each task

Camera

Phone numbers/ emails/ addresses

Reminders/ Task list

Dictaphone

Google Calendar
- Appointments
- Birthdays
- Social arrangements

Each evening, plan for day ahead:
- Check Google Calendar.
- Check to-do list.
- Reallocate any tasks not done.

Each morning, plan for that day:
- Check Google Calendar for what's coming up.
- Delete completed tasks immediately. If not, then delete the following morning.
- Get everything I need ready for the day.

Each week plan for week ahead:
- Check Google Calendar for upcoming week.
- Check to-do list and allocate times to tasks.

From *The Brain Injury Rehabilitation Workbook*, edited by Rachel Winson, Barbara A. Wilson, and Andrew Bateman. Copyright © 2017 The Guilford Press. Permission to photocopy this handout is granted to purchasers of this book for personal use or for use with individual clients (see copyright page for details). Purchasers can download additional copies of this handout (see the box at the end of the table of contents).

CHAPTER 5

Executive Functions

Jill Winegardner

"The term 'executive functions' refers to those abilities that enable a person to determine goals, formulate new and useful ways of achieving them, and then follow and adapt this proposed course in the face of competing demands and changing circumstances, often over long periods of time" (Burgess & Alderman, 2004, p. 185). Executive functions also involve the ability to regulate and control one's emotions and behavior. In addition, they are key to a person's awareness of and ability to recognize the changes produced by brain injury, especially changes in thinking, emotions, and behavior. Awareness is relevant to one's ability to recognize and perceive emotions both in oneself and in others.

This chapter aims to provide clinicians with tools to understand impairments of executive functions and learn strategies that can help clients manage these difficulties.

THEORETICAL BACKGROUND AND MODELS

Many models and theories have been developed to explain and clarify the nature of executive functions. The following discussion is not exhaustive, but provides brief descriptions of several prominent models.

Verbal Self-Regulation (Luria, 1966)

Luria wrote that frontal lobe injury results in a disturbance in the conscious and volitional self-regulation of behavior, so that people lose the ability to behave with intention. As a result, they may show decreased spontaneity or initiative. Luria believed that the loss of critical attitude toward one's own behavior causes problems in matching one's actions with the original intention.

Supervisory System (Shallice, 1981)

Shallice's model suggests that there are two levels of control. The first is routine control, which we develop by forming habits so that our responses become automatic. The second level is a higher level of voluntary, strategic control, which is the supervisory executive system. We use this system for planning and for recognizing and managing unforeseen consequences.

Goal Neglect Model (Duncan, 1986)

Normally we behave according to the presence of various internal goals; in other words, our behavior is driven by goals, and this makes the behavior predictable and directed. Executive dysfunction can disrupt the goal-driven nature of behavior, resulting in difficulty sustaining focus on a goal and in the ability to carry out the steps needed to reach the goal without getting distracted or going off target. A client with brain damage may know the right thing to do, but fail to do it.

Model of Frontal Lobe Functioning (Stuss, 2011)

The model proposed by Stuss provides evidence-based neuroanatomical linkage for four key domains of frontal lobe functioning. Although the model is intended to describe frontal lobe functioning, it is used here as a means of understanding executive functions in general. The model suggests that the four domains and their pathways are as follows:

1. Energization (or doing) domain
   - Showing energization and drive—getting started with tasks, staying engaged, and keeping up momentum.
   - Maintaining alertness and attention to tasks, and reacting at an appropriate speed.
   - Thinking things all the way through.
   - Having energy.
2. Executive cognition (or thinking) domain
   - Making and carrying out plans, staying on track, thinking flexibly, and switching from one task or idea to another.
   - Monitoring thoughts and actions.
   - Abstract thinking and problem solving.
3. Emotional and behavioral self-regulation (or feeling and acting) domain
   - Experiencing typical, predictable emotions that are appropriate to various situations.
   - Controlling emotions, thoughts, and actions appropriately.
   - Thinking things through before saying or doing them.
   - Showing mature emotional responsiveness.
4. Metacognition (or awareness and socializing) domain
   - Having an accurate understanding of the effects of a brain injury one has sustained.
   - Being aware of one's impact on other people.

- Seeing someone else's point of view and being sympathetic.
- Being able to read one's own emotions and the emotions of others.

NEUROANATOMY OF EXECUTIVE FUNCTIONS

In the Stuss model, the specific brain areas associated with the four domains are as follows:

1. Energization (doing): Dorsomedial cortex
2. Executive cognition (thinking): Dorsolateral prefrontal cortex (left: planning; right: monitoring)
3. Behavioral/emotional self-regulation (feeling and acting): Orbitofrontal cortex
4. Metacognition (awareness and socializing): Frontopolar region

The Stuss model is used in this chapter of this workbook because it provides a logical, complete, and intuitive approach to the understanding and management of executive functions for clients. The linkages between domains and brain areas are illustrated in Figures 5.1 and 5.2, and versions of these illustrations with simplified labels for clients are provided as Handouts 5.1 and 5.2, respectively.* The four domains have also been "translated" into everyday language in Handout 5.3, for the purposes of teaching clients about executive functions and of generating rehabilitation strategies based on the pattern of difficulties shown by each client.

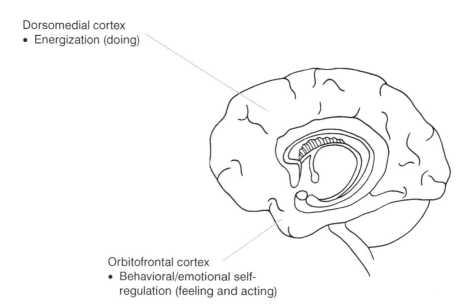

Dorsomedial cortex
• Energization (doing)

Orbitofrontal cortex
• Behavioral/emotional self-regulation (feeling and acting)

FIGURE 5.1. Brain areas involved in executive functions.

---

*All handouts appear at the end of the chapter.

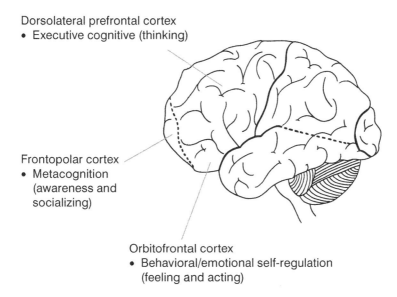

Dorsolateral prefrontal cortex
• Executive cognitive (thinking)

Frontopolar cortex
• Metacognition
  (awareness and
  socializing)

Orbitofrontal cortex
• Behavioral/emotional self-regulation
  (feeling and acting)

FIGURE 5.2. More brain areas involved in executive functions.

REHABILITATION: THE EVIDENCE

A growing evidence base exists for interventions to address executive dysfunctions. Kennedy et al. (2008) carried out a systematic review and meta-analysis that supported the use of metacognitive strategy instruction (MSI) for clients with traumatic brain injury (TBI). They concluded: "These results, along with positive outcomes from the other group, single-subject design and single-case studies, provided sufficient evidence to make the clinical recommendation that MSI should be used with young to middle-aged adults with TBI, when improvement in everyday, functional problems is the goal" (p. 257).

Cicerone et al. (2011, p. 523) provided another in a series of meta-analyses of the evidence base for cognitive rehabilitation and set out standards of care based on the significance of the evidence to date. For executive functions, their conclusions are as follows:

• *Practice Standard* (substantive evidence of effectiveness): Metacognitive strategy training (self-monitoring and self-regulation) is recommended for deficits in executive functioning after TBI, including impairments of emotional self-regulation, and as a component of interventions for deficits in attention, neglect, and memory.
• *Practice Guideline* (probable effectiveness): Training in formal problem-solving strategies and their application to everyday situations and functional activities is recommended during postacute rehabilitation after TBI.

More recently, an international team of researchers and clinicians collaborated as part of the INCOG project mentioned in earlier chapters to investigate evidence for management of executive dysfunction (Tate et al., 2014). They concluded:

Intervention programs incorporating metacognitive strategy instruction for planning, problem-solving, and other cognitive-executive impairments have a solid evidence base.

New evidence supports the use of strategies to specifically improve reasoning skills. Substantial support exists for use of direct corrective feedback to improve self-awareness. (p. 338)

EXPLORING EXECUTIVE FUNCTIONS AND DYSFUNCTIONS WITH CLIENTS

What Are Executive Functions?

Before considering strategies, you will need to help clients to understand what executive functions are and what kind of difficulties can occur following acquired brain injury. Handout 5.3, as noted above, offers simplified descriptions of the executive functions. Handout 5.4 asks clients to consider who needs good executive functions.

What Can Happen to Executive Functions after Brain Injury?

Handouts 5.5 and 5.6 focus on clients' experience of living with executive function problems and how these problems might be perceived by others around them. We highlight the concept that unlike other cognitive difficulties, executive dysfunctions can mirror personality flaws and are often misunderstood by clients and families alike. These handouts ask clients to reflect on their own executive function difficulties and help them understand that these are not due to personality features or to moral flaws, but rather to brain injury.

Handout 5.7 provides a story that illustrates ways in which executive functions have gone awry. Read the story to your clients and ask them to say "Bing!" every time they hear something that reflects a problem with executive functioning on the part of the writer. Alternatively, ask them to read the story and underline any phrases or words that suggest a problem with executive functions on the part of the writer.

Helping Clients Reflect on Executive Functions

The purpose of this exercise is to help clients reflect on their own and their peers' executive function patterns. Give each client five bowls and 20 beans. Four of the bowls should be marked with the names of the four domains ("Doing," "Thinking," "Feeling and Acting," and "Awareness and Socializing"), and the fifth bowl should be marked "None." Instruct clients to put beans in each bowl according to how much they perceive that particular domain as a problem for them. For example, someone who feels that he or she has the most problems with "Doing," and a bit of difficulty with "Thinking," but no problems with the other domains might put 14 beans in the "Doing" bowl and 6 beans in the "Thinking" bowl. Clients who feel they have no or few problems can put all or some of their beans in the "None" bowl.

Once the beans have been allotted to bowls, ask clients to tell the group why they allotted their beans as they have. Then ask the other group members to reflect on whether they agree or not with each client's allocation of beans.

ASSESSING EXECUTIVE FUNCTIONS

Assessing executive functions is very tricky for a number of reasons. First, executive functions are often considered a unitary construct rather than a complex of various underlying domains, so only one domain is tested. Most tests assess problems with executive cognitive abilities, such as planning, organizing, and flexible thinking. There are relatively few good tests of initiation, emotion regulation, and awareness in clinical use. Most test settings are highly structured and task initiation is prompted, so problems other than executive cognitive problems are likely to be missed.

Therefore, a good assessment of executive functions should include not only formal test results, but also behavioral observations; qualitative observations of functional activities; reports from family members and others; and questionnaires such as the Behavioural Assessment of the Dysexecutive Syndrome (Wilson, Emslie, Evans, Alderman, & Burgess, 1996) and the European Brain Injury Questionnaire (Teasdale et al., 1997).

REHABILITATION STRATEGIES

The choice of rehabilitation strategies needs to be based on each client's goals (see Wilson, Chapter 1, this volume) and on the nature of the client's executive functioning difficulties. The beans-and-bowls exercise described above is a good way to elicit clients' perceptions of the nature and the severity of their problems. This section describes a variety of strategies according to the domains of the Stuss model.

Strategies to Manage Energization Problems

Structured Routines

Routines can provide the necessary scaffolding to help clients follow a sequence of steps to reach a clearly stated goal. Routines should initially have as many steps and as much detail as needed for a client to be successful. Once the client can successfully follow the full routine, it is possible to begin combining steps and simplifying the structure. Each newly simplified routine should be used until the client is successful before it is again simplified. Some clients will continue to need fairly elaborate routines, while others will be able to reduce steps or eliminate routines once they have internalized them.

Here is an example of a structured morning routine for a client:

Goal: Be ready to go in the morning by 9:40 A.M.

Plan: Follow your text alerts; check the time you finish each step; do the steps in order.

NeuroPage messages the night before:

    10:30 P.M.: "Put meds, glass of water, and blood sugar equipment near alarm."

    10:45 P.M.: "Put meds and water in kitchen for after breakfast."

The morning routine:

- Step   1: Wake up to alarm placed far away, 7:15 A.M.
- Step   2: Take first meds, 7:20.
- Step   3: Drink large glass of water, 7:22.
- Step   4: Check blood sugar, 7:30.
- Step   5: Shower, 7:45.
- Step   6: Shave, 7:50.
- Step   7: Get dressed, 8:00.
- Step   8: Get contact lenses or glasses, 8:05.
- Step   9: Go down for breakfast, 8:10.
- Step 10: Take medications with water, 8:15.
- Step 11: Wash up after breakfast, 8:55.
- Step 12: Collect folder, phone, pens, and coat for the day, 9:25.
- Step 13: Check emails (optional, if time), 9:30.

Now review the routine!

Are things going well? If not, do you need to change your plan?

Alerts

Alerts can provide external reminders or stimuli to help "kick-start" a person with initiation problems into action. The advantages of alerts over getting reminders from other people are that clients can direct and plan the alerts themselves, and that personal relationships can be improved if families and caregivers have less reminding and nagging to do.

Clients who have smartphones and computers can learn to program their own alerts. Google Calendar has some evidence to support its use for prospective memory deficits (McDonald et al., 2011). Another system for alerts is NeuroPage (Wilson, Emslie, Quirk, & Evans, 2001), an evidence-based service that provides a pager to which messages are sent at predetermined times to facilitate independence for people with memory and executive functioning difficulties. Messages can also be sent to smartphones. Recent text-to-voice developments are ideal for those who cannot read.

Self-Instruction

The strategy of facilitating verbal mediation by teaching self-instruction to promote the internalization of verbal self-regulation was developed in response to Shallice's (1981) supervisory system model. Clients can be encouraged to use self-instruction techniques to prompt initiation and action.

The method involves prompting a client to state an instruction aloud first (e.g., "Take the dog for a walk now"), and to follow this by carrying out the action. The instruction is gradually internalized, so the next step is for the client to whisper the instruction and eventually to think it silently.

Management of Sleep Problems and Fatigue

Fatigue and sleep problems can have a significant negative impact on activation. For advice on managing fatigue, see Malley, Chapter 7, this volume.

Strategies to Manage Executive Cognition Problems

The strategies for memory and planning systems described by Fish and Brentnall (Chapter 4, this volume) may also be useful for planning difficulties that are due to executive dysfunction.

Stop/Think

"Stop/Think" is an informal technique to encourage clients to pause and reflect on their intentions before implementing them. Accordingly, it is a helpful tool for managing impulsivity, as well as for improving planning and decision making. The use of Stop/Think can be incorporated into other strategies discussed, such as Time Pressure Management (TPM) or the Goal Management Framework (GMF); it can also be used as a mood-monitoring strategy.

Clients can be reminded to use Stop/Think both within and outside sessions, and to use Handout 5.8 for actively monitoring their use of the strategy until it becomes a habit.

Zoom In/Out

The "Zoom In/Out" strategy addresses problems with abstract thinking that manifest themselves as difficulty with thinking at the right level of detail. This problem may involve a tendency to think too broadly and globally, resulting in being overly abstract, or too narrowly, resulting in difficulty seeing the bigger picture. The strategy therefore centers on the importance of being able to move flexibly between thinking broadly and focusing on details, as needed. People with problems in executive functioning often find it difficult to use both of these ways of thinking.

The Zoom In/Out strategy involves encouraging clients to expand their focus beyond the most concrete level to include a bigger circle of awareness. For example, clients may be asked to think beyond the current moment into the future and to take future consequences of current behavior into consideration, or they may be asked to expand their concern beyond themselves to include the views and feelings of other persons.

To help clients practice choosing the right level of focus to solve a problem, play a version of the well-known game of Twenty Questions. Think of a famous person who will be well known to all present. The clients are to find out who it is by asking questions that can only be answered by "Yes" or "No." Clients are encouraged first to consider broad and general questions, and then to narrow in on the details once they have established the general parameters. For example, ideally they will start with asking whether the person is male or female and living or dead, and then move on to categories such as general age, location, and broad professional identity before narrowing in on specific jobs or names. Ask the clients to choose their questions as a group in order to facilitate a thoughtful process.

These rules should be written on a flip chart or board so that everyone can refer to them as needed. Write up the answers so that they can be reviewed periodically.

Time Pressure Management

TPM (Fasotti, Kovacs, Eling, & Brouwer, 2000) is a cognitive strategy designed to help people with brain injury and slowed information processing manage tasks in a way that reduces the time pressure on them to complete these tasks, and therefore improves their success rate and reduces their stress. Basically, TPM is a way for such people to make sure they have enough time to complete a given task successfully. TPM is particularly useful for clients with executive functioning difficulties as a tool to improve planning, organization, and decision making. It can help such clients to become more aware of the steps that are needed and to think through a task in an orderly way. It can also help make them more aware of everything that will be needed to complete the task. And it can help to prevent potential problems with time pressure and to manage them when they do occur.

TPM involves breaking a task down into elements that can be handled at three different levels: "strategic," "tactical," and "operational." Time pressure typically occurs if a person has not allotted enough time for a task, considered potential things that could go wrong, or thought through alternatives in case of emergency at the beginning. By thinking ahead strategically about the plan, a client should be better able to avoid these problems.

Fasotti et al.'s TPM protocol uses the following steps:

1. Are there two or more things to be done at the same time for which there is not enough time? If yes, go to Step 2; otherwise, just do the task. (Awareness of time pressure.)
2. Make a short plan of which things can be done before the actual task begins. (Planning to prevent time pressure.)
3. Make an emergency plan describing what to do in case of overwhelming time pressure. (Managing time pressure as quickly and effectively as possible.)
4. Are the plan and emergency plan ready? Then use them regularly as needed! (Monitoring.)

Have clients practice TPM by setting them the task of preparing a meal consisting of three items (main course, vegetable side dish, and dessert). Before they begin, ask them to consider the following questions, generating as many ideas as they can:

- *What problems could create a time pressure crisis (planning level)?* Some examples may include forgetting to buy all the ingredients ahead of time; being unaware of the cooking time that is needed; needing extra time to prepare the ingredients; not having all the necessary utensils or equipment; finding that the stovetop or oven is failing to work properly; having trouble paying attention to two things at once; or starting at the last minute.

- *What can be done ahead of time to avoid time pressure problems (strategic level)?*
- *What can be done during the preparation of the ingredients to avoid time pressure problems (tactical level)?*
- *What can be done in the last minutes of cooking to avoid time pressure problems (operational level)?*

Goal Management Framework

The GMF is another tool for planning, making decisions, reaching goals, and problem solving. Today there are many forms of the GMF in use, but it is based on the work of Levine et al. (2000). The GMF can be applied in many settings, including business and management; its use need not be specific to clients with brain injury.

The version used at The Oliver Zangwill Centre and described here has six steps:

1. *Set the main goal.* Carefully identifying a client's main goal is very important, as it keeps the client on the right track to achieve it. The main goal needs to be as specific as possible.

2. *Identify possible solutions.* This step involves generating as many solutions to reach the goal as possible. Encourage clients to "think outside the box" and to include even silly ideas, as a way to encourage creativity and push those who struggle to generate ideas.

3. *Weigh up pros and cons.* This step requires weighing up the good points and the bad points of each option identified in Step 2 for achieving the main goal. It is important to evaluate not just the number of pros and cons, but also the relative weights of each. (For example, a goal might be to purchase a new car, and the options may include a Jaguar; however, the expense of a Jaguar may outweigh the pleasure of driving it.)

4. *Choose a solution and plan the steps.* The client then chooses one of the options, based on the analysis of the good and bad points and their relative weights. Next, the client plans the steps needed to achieve the goal. This planning includes listing the steps in the proper sequence as well as noting other strategies that might be useful. Ask clients, and encourage clients to ask themselves, these questions:

- What are the steps?
- In what order should the steps be carried out?
- What other strategies can be used?

5. *Do it!* In this step, the client follows the plan and implements the actions identified in earlier steps. Clients may need support to check in with themselves. Ask clients, and encourage them to ask themselves, these questions:

- Are you following your plan?
- Are you doing the right step?
- How are you going to make sure that you are on track?

6. *Monitor and evaluate progress.* It is important to engage clients in reflecting on their choices and actions throughout the implementation of the plan. This process strengthens the habit of self-monitoring and can reduce impulsivity. Here are some questions to ask clients, and for clients to ask themselves:

- Reflect on what you learned from the task.
- Could you have done anything differently?
- What did you do especially well?

Once clients have been introduced to the GMF, present the following dilemma to the clients, and ask them to use the GMF to solve it and to work as a group:

"It's early evening. You have a group of friends coming over for dinner. You've spent the weekly shopping money on the meal. You start preparing the meal and find that the oven doesn't work. Your landlord had said he would replace your oven next week. The guests arrive in 2 hours. What do you do?"

Now support clients to use Handout 5.9 to execute the GMF.

Memory Strategies

Strategies that support memory difficulties can also be useful for executive cognitive problems. For example, the mental blackboard can be used to reduce goal neglect and improve maintenance of focus by helping a client to keep the main goal in mind. See Fish and Brentnall, Chapter 4, this volume, for further suggestions.

Cue Cards

Clients may benefit from wallet-sized laminated cue cards that contain reminders for any of the strategies that are most useful to them. Handout 5.10 offers two examples; you can also encourage clients to create their own.

Strategies to Manage Emotional/Behavioral Dyscontrol

There are three key steps in managing emotional and behavioral dysregulation following brain injury: understanding the nature of the problems; recognizing early signs of rising emotions; and using calming strategies.

Understanding the Problems

Behavioral and emotional dysregulation are extremely distressing experiences, both for people with the injury and for those around them. The essential first step in helping clients manage these problems, therefore, is psychoeducation about the nature of emotional and behavioral changes following brain injury. Use the information provided by Ford in Chapter 8 of this volume to help the clients understand these changes.

Recognizing Early Signs of Rising Emotions

Once clients understand the reasons for changes in their ability to control and regulate their emotions and behavior, help them learn to recognize their own early warning signs. The emotion thermometer illustrated in Handout 5.11 can support understanding of how emotions can quickly get out of control. As well as being used to notice symptoms of fatigue, the gingerbread person depicted in Handout 7.8 (see Malley, Chapter 7, this volume) can be used to help clients notice physical changes in their bodies when they are becoming angry.

Another tool that is useful for helping clients who have difficulty in recognizing internal sensations is the Actiheart. The Actiheart is a monitoring device that records heart rate and interbeat interval (Brage et al., 2005). It clips onto two electrocardiographic electrodes worn on the chest; it is compact, lightweight, waterproof, and noninvasive. The Actiheart provides biofeedback so that a client can recognize when his or her heart rate is rising and can correlate this with emotional triggers.

Using Calming Strategies

Once clients understand why their emotions are difficult to control and can recognize signs of rising emotions, it is time to teach the use of calming strategies. Both cognitive and mood-oriented strategies can be useful. For example, teaching clients to use Stop/Think provides them with a prompt to use their thinking skills when they feel an emotional reaction, thus engaging their frontal-lobe-based logic and reasoning abilities. Use of the GMF can help clients contemplate various alternative reasons for situations that anger them, and then devise a variety of responses in addition to immediate, emotionally driven responses. Calming strategies are most useful when practiced in advance, so that they become habitual and readily available for use at times of need. Chapter 8 on mood introduces different calming strategies, each of which has a different mode of working. These strategies can be presented as "samples" to clients, who can then choose those they like most to continue practicing.

Strategies to Manage Metacognition and Awareness Problems

Problems with metacognition and awareness create serious barriers to change for clients and contribute greatly to interpersonal disruptions. They can also be the most difficult problems to treat, for the very reason that the clients may not see the need for change and therefore may not think that increased awareness and sensitivity to others are needed as goals.

Zoom In/Out

In addition to supporting executive cognition, the Zoom In/Out strategy is relevant for improving awareness and sensitivity because it helps clients think beyond their own immediate concerns and needs to the future implications of their actions. It can also help them expand their circles of concern to include other people and their feelings.

Feedback

Feedback can come from others—both other clients and staff members. One major advantage of working with groups is the opportunity for clients to give one another valuable feedback in a "safe" setting. Hearing feedback from other clients can be much more powerful and effective than feedback from staff or family members.

There is some evidence base for interventions designed to improve clients' awareness of their own behaviors and sensitivity to others. Video feedback has been found to be more effective than verbal feedback (Schmidt, Fleming, Ownsworth, & Lannin, 2013), and there is some moderate evidence for the general effectiveness of using feedback to address lack of awareness (Schmidt, Lannin, Fleming, & Ownsworth, 2011).

Giving feedback must be done carefully and should always include both strengths and challenges. It should also include options for making changes to problematic behaviors, ideally with opportunities to practice the new behaviors. Feedback should be both immediate and direct whenever possible. In groups, it may not be possible to give feedback in front of others, so help clients decide ahead of time how they wish to receive their feedback. A client might be comfortable with direct feedback in a group setting, might prefer to receive the feedback in private immediately after the group ends, or might choose to receive a sign from you (the therapist) indicating that a behavior has taken place. For example, you and a client might agree that if the client shouts in a group, you will signal this to the client by putting a hand to your ear.

Behavioral Experiments

Behavioral experiments were developed as a component of cognitive-behavioral therapy for the purpose of helping clients identify and challenge negative beliefs (Bennett-Levy et al., 2004). A client identifies a negative or maladaptive belief, such as "Only people with brain . injuries use lists to support their memory problems." The belief is then challenged through an experiment in which the client predicts the outcome and plans the experiment. In this example, the client might predict that none of the staff members of a brain injury program use lists to remember things. Then the client might design a short survey and give it to all of the staff members. Results are reviewed to see whether they support the predictions or not, and if they do not, the old beliefs are challenged and discarded. In this example, learning that many people without brain injuries use lists as memory aids may help normalize the strategy and make it more acceptable to the client.

Behavioral experiments can be designed for clients who have metacognitive difficulties to help them develop more realistic beliefs about themselves while supporting them to see the benefits of using strategies. Handout 5.12 can be used to facilitate the development and use of such experiments. The following questions may help to guide a client's predictions and reflections:

- In this situation, what do you think might happen?
- How do you think you will feel?

- How do you think you will respond?
- Do you feel you have the abilities needed to do this task?
- Do you feel your efforts will result in achievement?
- Is this task important for you?
- Will you enjoy doing this activity? Why/why not?
- What skills (cognitive, motor, and/or communicative) will facilitate/restrict your performance?
- How might the environment help or hinder you in reaching your goal?

Ford (Chapter 8, this volume) offers more guidance on using behavioral experiments.

BRINGING IT ALL TOGETHER

The next exercise is designed for use after all of the executive function strategies described above have been taught and practiced. It works well in a group context or with individual clients, and can be modified to fit the needs of different settings.

In a group, allocate roles such as leader, note taker, budget manager, time keeper, and observer. Roles can be assigned to clients that are outside of their comfort zones. For example, a client who is domineering and tends to interrupt may be assigned the role of observer, while a shy client might be asked to be group leader. Observe the process, and remind the group to use both cognitive and calming strategies in order to facilitate a good outcome.

Next, ask clients to create a buffet lunch for themselves plus the group facilitators, using all the strategies they have learned so far. Provide them with these sets of "rules" and "freedoms":

Rules
Include both hot and cold items in the buffet.
You should have one sweet item.
You may need to take into account any dietary requirements or allergies of guests.
Your budget is £25/$40 (or the equivalent of about £5/$8 per person).
You have a time limit (to be determined by the group facilitators).

Freedoms
You may include any items that you wish in the buffet.
You may buy items for the buffet from anywhere you wish.

In a community setting, the activity could be adapted to involve the clients' preparing a multicomponent meal for friends or family members.

COMPLETING AN EXECUTIVE FUNCTION PROFILE

Clients may wish to complete a copy of the executive function profile sheet (Handout 5.13) to add to their portfolios. Use the information gathered from monitoring sheets and activities to help clients identify their strengths and challenges with regard to executive functions, along with any factors relating to attention and memory that affect executive functioning, and helpful strategies for meeting the challenges.

CASE STUDY

The case of Jeff, whose severe TBI in a traffic accident at age 19 cut short his plans for accepting a golf scholarship in the United States, has been introduced by Fish and colleagues at the end of Chapter 3. The problems Jeff faced with regard to executive functions and some of his goals and strategies for dealing with these problems, are described in Table 5.1.

TABLE 5.1. Dealing with Jeff's Executive Functioning Challenges

Challenges	Goals and strategies	Context for rehabilitation
Energization Jeff had difficulty generating and elaborating ideas. He also showed poor initiative and carry-through of plans outside his fixed routine. For instance, Jeff wanted to work as a golf tutor, but he struggled to come up with ideas for lessons and exercises.	Goals: To find voluntary/paid work as a golf tutor. Cognitive strategies: • Stop/Think • GMF Mood management strategies: • Compassion-focused therapy • Calming breathing • Mindfulness	Jeff was supported to plan and deliver golf lessons to staff and fellow clients. To build awareness, Jeff gave a golf lesson without any prior planning, and got feedback from his students. The session lacked structure and content.
Executive cognition Jeff showed limited flexible thinking, was impulsive, and had difficulty monitoring his thoughts and actions. For instance, he once corrected a student's stance by striking him behind the knees with a golf club.	Techniques for building awareness: • Video feedback • Psychoeducation • Monitoring and feedback from staff and peers	He was supported to use a set structure for lesson planning. This was initially done with guidance, which was reduced over time until he was able to plan a lesson independently using a template.
Behavioral/emotional self-regulation Jeff was irritable and verbally aggressive, and, again, he had problems monitoring and evaluating his behaviors. For instance, he was constantly snapping at his family out of frustration.		Short phrases, mnemonics, and analogies were used to support planning and explanation of techniques to students. Jeff used Stop/Think to check that he had enough content prior to the lesson, and also to monitor communication in lessons. GMF was used to support decision making.
Metacognition Jeff's awareness of his deficits was fluctuating and superficial. He was unable to make the connections between his life problems and his brain-injury-related impairments. For instance, he could not understand why he was no longer welcome at his old golf club following incidents of inappropriate behavior, as he was still a good golfer.		Jeff built a library of exercises to use in future sessions and created a portfolio of lesson plans to use when applying for volunteer coaching positions at his local golf club.

REFERENCES

Bennett-Levy, J., Butler, G., Fennell, M., Hackmann, A., Mueller, M., & Westbrook, D. (Eds.). (2004). *Oxford guide to behavioural experiments in cognitive therapy.* Oxford, UK: Oxford University Press.

Brage, S., Brage, N., Franks, P. W., Ekelund, U., & Wareham, N. J. (2005). Reliability and validity of the combined heart rate and movement sensor Actiheart. *European Journal of Clinical Nutrition, 59*(4), 561–570.

Burgess, P. W., & Alderman, N. (2004). Executive dysfunction. In L. H. Goldstein & J. E. McNeil (Eds.), *Clinical neuropsychology: A practical guide to assessment and management for clinicians* (pp. 185–210). Chichester, UK: Wiley.

Cicerone, K. D. (2002). The enigma of executive functioning: Theoretical contributions to therapeutic interventions. In P. J. Eslinger (Ed.), *Neuropsychological interventions: Clinical research and practice* (pp. 246–265). New York: Guilford Press.

Cicerone, K. D., Langenbahn, D. M., Braden, C., Malec, J. F., Kalmar, K., Fraas, M., . . . Ashman, T. (2011). Evidence-based cognitive rehabilitation: Updated review of the literature from 2003 through 2008. *Archives of Physical Medicine and Rehabilitation, 92*(4), 519–530.

Duncan, J. (1986). Disorganisation of behavior after frontal lobe damage. *Cognitive Neuropsychology, 3*(3), 271–290.

Fasotti, L., Kovacs, F., Eling, P., & Brouwer, W. (2000). Time pressure management as a compensatory strategy training after closed head injury. *Neuropsychological Rehabilitation, 10*(1), 47–65.

Kennedy, M. R., Coelho, C., Turkstra, L., Ylvisaker, M., Moore Sohlberg, M., Yorkston, K., . . . Kan, P. F. (2008). Intervention for executive functions after traumatic brain injury: A systematic review, meta-analysis and clinical recommendations. *Neuropsychological Rehabilitation, 18*(3), 257–299.

Levine, B., Robertson, I. H., Clare, L., Carter, G., Hong, J., Wilson, B. A., . . . Stuss, D. T. (2000). Rehabilitation of executive functioning: An experimental-clinical validation of goal management training. *Journal of the International Neuropsychological Society, 6*(3), 299–312.

Luria, A. R. (1966). *Higher cortical functions in man.* New York: Basic Books.

McDonald, A., Haslam, C., Yates, P., Gurr, B., Leeder, G., & Sayers, A. (2011). Google calendar: A new memory aid to compensate for prospective memory deficits following acquired brain injury. *Neuropsychological Rehabilitation, 21*(6), 784–807.

Schmidt, J., Fleming, J., Ownsworth, T., & Lannin, N. (2013). Videotape feedback on functional task performance improves self-awareness after traumatic brain injury: A randomized controlled trial. *Journal of Neurorehabilitation and Neural Repair, 27,* 316–324.

Schmidt, J., Lannin, N., Fleming, J., & Ownsworth, T. (2011). Feedback interventions for impaired self-awareness following brain injury: A systematic review. *Journal of Rehabilitation Medicine, 43*(8), 673–680.

Shallice, T. (1981). Neurological impairment of cognitive processes. *British Medical Bulletin, 37*(2), 187–192.

Stuss, D. T. (2011). Traumatic brain injury: Relation to executive dysfunction and the frontal lobes. *Current Opinion in Neurology, 24*(6), 584–589.

Tate, R., Kennedy, M., Ponsford, J., Douglas, J., Velikonja, D., Bayley, M., & Stergiou-Kita, M. (2014). INCOG recommendations for management of cognition following traumatic brain injury: Part III. Executive function and self-awareness. *Journal of Head Trauma Rehabilitation, 29*(4), 338–352.

Teasdale, T. W., Christensen, A. L., Willmes, K., Deloche, G., Braga, L., Stachowiak, F., . . . &

Leclercq, M. (1997). Subjective experience in brain-injured patients and their close relatives: A European Brain Injury Questionnaire study. *Brain Injury, 11*(8), 543–564.

Wilson, B. A., Emslie, H., Evans, J. J., Alderman, N., & Burgess, P. W. (1996). *Behavioural Assessment of the Dysexecutive Syndrome.* London: Pearson.

Wilson, B. A., Emslie, H. C., Quirk, K., & Evans, J. J. (2001). Reducing everyday memory and planning problems by means of a paging system: A randomized control crossover study. *Journal of Neurology, Neurosurgery and Psychiatry, 70*(4), 477–482.

Brain Areas Involved in Executive Functions

It's important to remember that all parts of the brain work together; however, the areas shown here are active when we do complex tasks involving goal setting, planning, and monitoring.

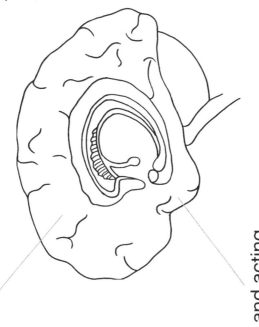

Getting started and doing

Feeling and acting

From *The Brain Injury Rehabilitation Workbook*, edited by Rachel Winson, Barbara A. Wilson, and Andrew Bateman. Copyright © 2017 The Guilford Press. Permission to photocopy this handout is granted to purchasers of this book for personal use or for use with individual clients (see copyright page for details). Purchasers can download additional copies of this handout (see the box at the end of the table of contents).

More Brain Areas Involved in Executive Functions

It's important to remember that all parts of the brain work together; however, the areas shown here are active when we do complex tasks involving goal setting, planning, and monitoring.

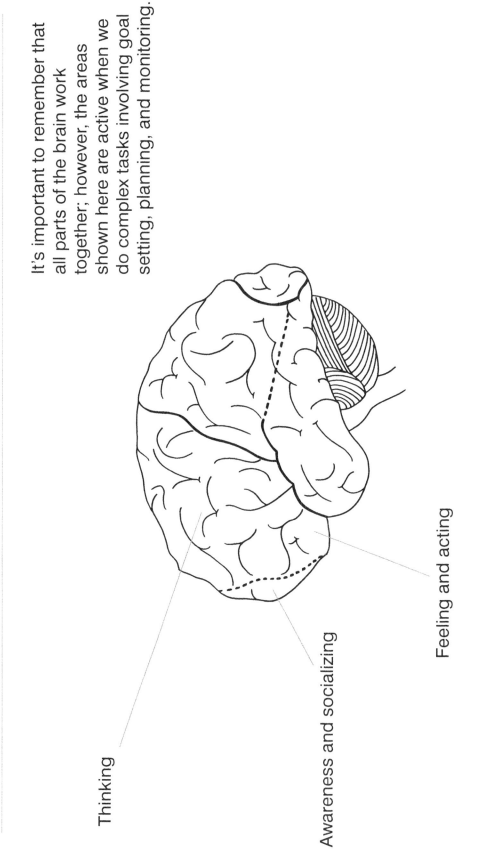

Thinking

Awareness and socializing

Feeling and acting

From *The Brain Injury Rehabilitation Workbook*, edited by Rachel Winson, Barbara A. Wilson, and Andrew Bateman. Copyright © 2017 The Guilford Press. Permission to photocopy this handout is granted to purchasers of this book for personal use or for use with individual clients (see copyright page for details). Purchasers can download additional copies of this handout (see the box at the end of the table of contents).

What Are Executive Functions?

The four domains of executive functions can be described in these simple terms:

Energization—*doing*

Executive cognition—*thinking*

Emotional and behavioral self-regulation—*feeling and acting*

Metacognition—*awareness and socializing*

The energization (doing) domain involves these abilities:

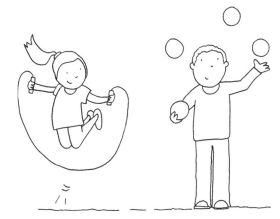

Ability to show activation and drive.

Alertness.

Maintaining attention to tasks.

Normal reaction speed.

Thinking things all the way through.

Maintaining momentum.

Ease in getting started with things.

Staying engaged.

Staying interested.

Having energy.

The executive cognition (thinking) domain involves these abilities:

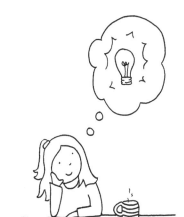

Making and carrying out plans.

Staying on track.

Monitoring thoughts and actions.

Switching from one task or idea to another.

Thinking flexibly.

Abstract thinking.

Problem solving.

(continued)

From *The Brain Injury Rehabilitation Workbook*, edited by Rachel Winson, Barbara A. Wilson, and Andrew Bateman. Copyright © 2017 The Guilford Press. Permission to photocopy this handout is granted to purchasers of this book for personal use or for use with individual clients (see copyright page for details). Purchasers can download additional copies of this handout (see the box at the end of the table of contents).

The emotional and behavioral self-regulation (feeling and acting) domain involves these abilities:

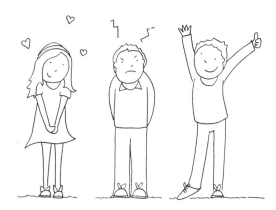

Experiencing typical emotions in response to various situations.

Experiencing emotions that fit the situation and are predictable.

Controlling emotions appropriately.

Controlling thoughts and actions.

Thinking things through before saying or doing them.

Showing mature emotional responsiveness.

The metacognition (awareness and socializing) domain involves these abilities:

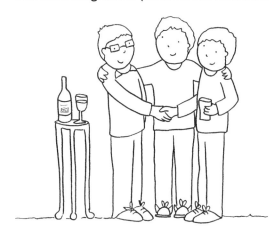

Having an accurate understanding of how your brain injury has affected you.

Being aware of your impact on other people.

Being able to take someone else's point of view.

Being sympathetic to someone else.

Being able to read your own emotions.

Being able to read someone else's emotions.

Who Needs Good Executive Functions?

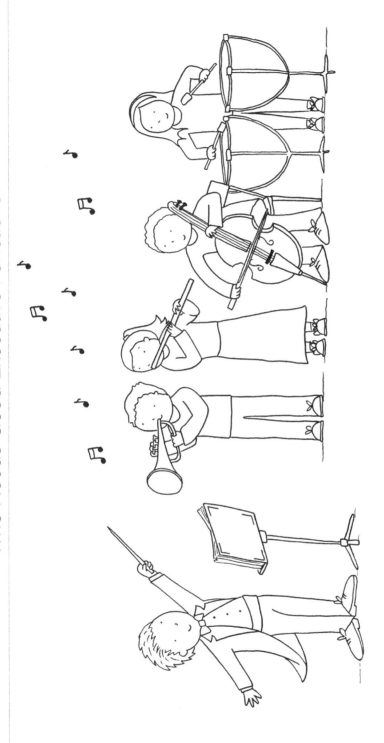

An orchestra conductor!

- The conductor has to *plan* the concert, *select* the music, *organize* the musicians, *start* the music, *make decisions* during the performance, *monitor* the overall sound, *solve any problems* during the performance, and *keep the main goal in mind!*

Who else needs good executive functions?

- You do!
- Can you think of examples where you need good executive functions in your own life?

From *The Brain Injury Rehabilitation Workbook*, edited by Rachel Winson, Barbara A. Wilson, and Andrew Bateman. Copyright © 2017 The Guilford Press. Permission to photocopy this handout is granted to purchasers of this book for personal use or for use with individual clients (see copyright page for details). Purchasers can download additional copies of this handout (see the box at the end of the table of contents).

How Does It Feel?

Executive function problems often get confused with personality problems.
Let's go through them in more detail.

Energization (Doing)

What does it feel like to the person who experiences problems with energization and drive?

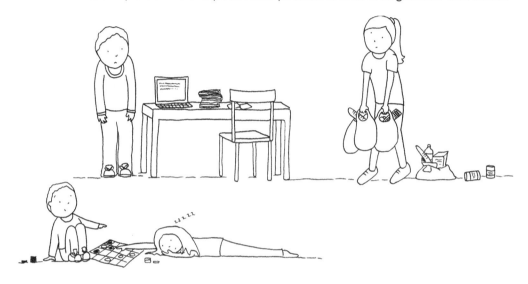

"I have no energy."

"I get bored so easily."

"I am just really slow."

"It is hard to get started with things."

"It is hard to keep going even after I get started."

"It is difficult to stay engaged."

"Do I just not care any more?"

What do these problems look like to other people?

"She seems to be lazy now, lacking any motivation. She needs to be made to do things."

(continued)

From *The Brain Injury Rehabilitation Workbook*, edited by Rachel Winson, Barbara A. Wilson, and Andrew Bateman. Copyright © 2017 The Guilford Press. Permission to photocopy this handout is granted to purchasers of this book for personal use or for use with individual clients (see copyright page for details). Purchasers can download additional copies of this handout (see the box at the end of the table of contents).

Executive Cognition (Thinking)

What do problems with thinking feel like?

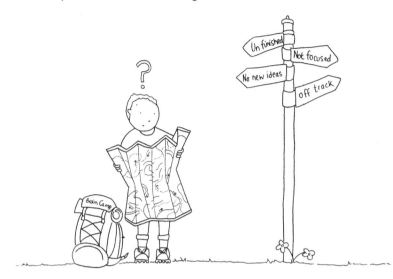

"I have trouble coming up with new ideas."

"It's easy to go off track and not get back on target."

"It's hard to get things finished."

"I can't stick with a plan or an idea."

"It is difficult to solve problems."

"I can't really think outside the box."

"Am I just stupid now?"

What do these problems look like to other people?

"She's so repetitive. She'll get stuck on one topic of conversation when everyone else has moved on."

"She won't take advice, but insists on trying to do things her own way, even when it clearly isn't working."

"Since his head injury, my son has difficulty understanding anything subtle or abstract. He takes things very literally and is unable to see another point of view. He's so rigid."

How Does It Feel? (Continued)

Let's continue going through executive function problems and noting how they often get confused with personality problems.

Emotional and Behavioral Self-Regulation (Feeling and Acting)

What do problems with emotions and behaviors feel like?

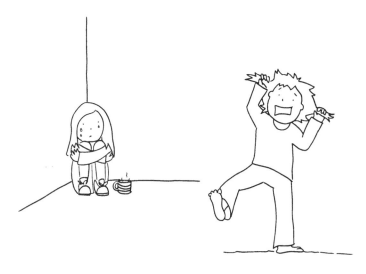

"I feel out of control."

"Emotions rise up way too quickly."

"I get emotional—out of the blue!"

"I can't predict what I will do or say."

"I might have anger outbursts, or cry for no good reason, or laugh when I don't want to."

"I'm embarrassing myself."

"I hate being rude or mean to other people."

"I'm impulsive."

"I say or do things without thinking them through."

"Have I become an out-of-control jerk?"

What do these problems look like to other people?

"He says and does things that are quite rude, and very out of character for him. He seems to do these things without thinking."

"She seems childish and selfish now."

(continued)

From *The Brain Injury Rehabilitation Workbook*, edited by Rachel Winson, Barbara A. Wilson, and Andrew Bateman. Copyright © 2017 The Guilford Press. Permission to photocopy this handout is granted to purchasers of this book for personal use or for use with individual clients (see copyright page for details). Purchasers can download additional copies of this handout (see the box at the end of the table of contents).

Metacognition (Awareness and Socializing)

What do problems with awareness and socializing feel like?

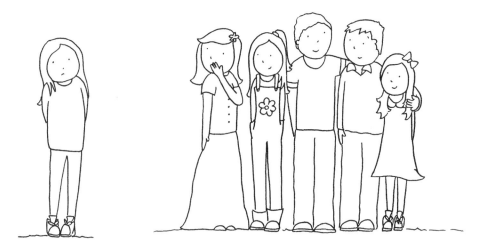

"Other people keep saying I have changed, but I feel like the same old me."

"It's harder to get along with other people now."

"I've lost friends and even some family members."

"Could there be something wrong that I don't know about, or is it them?"

What do these problems look like to other people?

"He is a completely different person now, and he doesn't even know it."

Christmas at JFK Airport

Read the story and highlight the executive functioning problems.

On December 22, 1987, I departed for New York. The journey was going to be characteristic for the way I arrange things. The trouble started a few days before the departure. I did not have the time to get a visa for the United States. But the American Embassy in Copenhagen has a fast procedure; 27 minutes was all it took to get a visa. Still, the problem was that the embassy did not open until 9:00 A.M., so I had a time crunch: I had to be at the airport at 9:50 A.M., and so I had to take a taxi to the airport. Doing this, I spent all the money that I had brought along for the trip. But I did not consider this a big problem, believing that my parents were going to meet me at the airport.

When the airplane arrived in New York, I decided to go to my parents' address in New York by bus and taxi. But having no money left, I was forced to figure out some alternative plan. My thoughts went like this: "If I do not show up at my parents' address, they will know something went wrong. The first thing they would do would be to check my home address in Copenhagen. The people at my home address would tell my parents that I had departed for New York. The next thing my parents would do would be to check with the airline in order to know if I had actually departed." I was wrong, however. At my home address, they were convinced that I had not had the time to get a visa, and for some reason the airline's computer had not registered my name.

Knowing nothing about these problems, I sat down and waited outside at the airport terminal. The terminal's outside waiting area closed at 11:00 P.M., so I had to find another place to spend the night. I stayed in the internal terminal, which is open 24 hours a day. I woke the next morning at 9:00 A.M. and I was wondering what to do, and finally decided to read a book. Actually, I did not do much this day (or any of the other days) except read a lot. The next day (the day of disappointments), December 24, nothing happened. Now that Christmas Eve had passed, I had given up hope of being picked up. I did not really know what to do next, so I continued to sit there and think things over. This did not help me, no matter how much I thought.

My parents were not in New York after December 24. So I started waiting for my departure for Denmark. The problem was that I had a ticket that could only be used for one fixed departure, and was impossible to change. In other words, I could not get anywhere until January 4. The days went by; I spent my time reading, walking around, or just sitting. I slept, I walked around, or I sat down thinking about life and its endless struggle. However, I had nowhere to go, so there was not much of a choice.

On January 4, I could finally use my ticket again, and so I departed for Denmark. I had lost weight, but gained much experience (or cautiousness) when I returned to Denmark. Being able to spend money again, the first thing I did was to buy myself a hot dog. I never knew they could taste that good.

Modified from A. Christensen (personal communication, 1987).

From *The Brain Injury Rehabilitation Workbook*, edited by Rachel Winson, Barbara A. Wilson, and Andrew Bateman. Copyright © 2017 The Guilford Press. Permission to photocopy this handout is granted to purchasers of this book for personal use or for use with individual clients (see copyright page for details). Purchasers can download additional copies of this handout (see the box at the end of the table of contents).

HANDOUT 5.8

Monitoring My Use of Stop/Think

Date/time	Trigger	Did I use Stop/Think?	Reflection

From *The Brain Injury Rehabilitation Workbook*, edited by Rachel Winson, Barbara A. Wilson, and Andrew Bateman. Copyright © 2017 The Guilford Press. Permission to photocopy this handout is granted to purchasers of this book for personal use or for use with individual clients (see copyright page for details). Purchasers can download additional copies of this handout (see the box at the end of the table of contents).

Using the Goal Management Framework (GMF)

1. What is the main goal?
   Stop/Think!

2. List all possible solutions. Think outside the box.
   Stop/Think!

3. Weigh up the pros and cons.

Possible solutions	Pros	Cons

   Stop/Think!

4. Choose a solution, and then plan the steps. Use your strategies.

   Step 1: _____

   Step 2: _____

   Step 3: _____

   Step 4: _____

   Step 5: _____

5. Do it!

6. Now review it! Are things going well? If not, do you need to change your plan?

From *The Brain Injury Rehabilitation Workbook*, edited by Rachel Winson, Barbara A. Wilson, and Andrew Bateman. Copyright © 2017 The Guilford Press. Permission to photocopy this handout is granted to purchasers of this book for personal use or for use with individual clients (see copyright page for details). Purchasers can download additional copies of this handout (see the box at the end of the table of contents).

Cue Cards

Goal Management Framework (GMF)

1. What is my goal? (*What am I trying to achieve?*)
2. Identify the possible solutions. (*Think outside the box!*)
3. Weigh up the pros and cons.
4. Make a decision and plan the steps.
5. Do it!
6. Review it and evaluate.

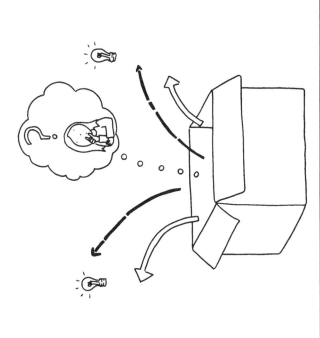

Stop/Think!

Take a calming breath.

Slow down the pace.

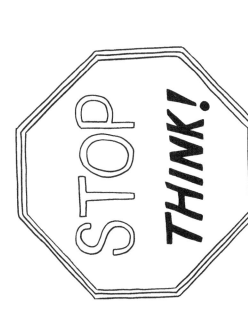

From *The Brain Injury Rehabilitation Workbook*, edited by Rachel Winson, Barbara A. Wilson, and Andrew Bateman. Copyright © 2017 The Guilford Press. Permission to photocopy this handout is granted to purchasers of this book for personal use or for use with individual clients (see copyright page for details). Purchasers can download additional copies of this handout (see the box at the end of the table of contents).

Emotion Thermometer

- Following brain injury, changes in emotion can be much more rapid.
- These changes in emotion can make it harder for us to think and solve problems.
- Tracking our emotions, as if we were measuring our temperature, can help us to manage our feelings before we get to boiling point.

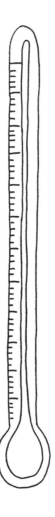

From *The Brain Injury Rehabilitation Workbook*, edited by Rachel Winson, Barbara A. Wilson, and Andrew Bateman. Copyright © 2017 The Guilford Press. Permission to photocopy this handout is granted to purchasers of this book for personal use or for use with individual clients (see copyright page for details). Purchasers can download additional copies of this handout (see the box at the end of the table of contents).

Behavioral Experiment

Experiment: Plan the task.	Predictions: What do you think will happen?	What happened?	Reflection: Were your predictions correct? What would you change next time?

From *The Brain Injury Rehabilitation Workbook*, edited by Rachel Winson, Barbara A. Wilson, and Andrew Bateman. Copyright © 2017 The Guilford Press. Permission to photocopy this handout is granted to purchasers of this book for personal use or for use with individual clients (see copyright page for details). Purchasers can download additional copies of this handout (see the box at the end of the table of contents).

My Executive Functioning Profile

When do I need to use executive functions?	
Executive functions that are strengths for me	
Executive functions that are challenges for me	
Which strategies work?	
How do my attention and memory affect my executive functions?	
What next?	

From *The Brain Injury Rehabilitation Workbook*, edited by Rachel Winson, Barbara A. Wilson, and Andrew Bateman. Copyright © 2017 The Guilford Press. Permission to photocopy this handout is granted to purchasers of this book for personal use or for use with individual clients (see copyright page for details). Purchasers can download additional copies of this handout (see the box at the end of the table of contents).

CHAPTER 6

Communication

Clare Keohane
Leyla Prince

Communication abilities are thought to play a pivotal role in determining quality of life after acquired brain injury (ABI). According to Struchen et al. (2008), impairments in communication following traumatic brain injury (TBI) are becoming increasingly recognized as significant factors in reconstructing identity, resuming former life roles, returning to work, adapting psychosocially, and forming and maintaining relationships. Social isolation as a consequence of impaired social interaction has been reported as one of the most common and devastating sequelae of TBI; it has a negative impact on families as well as individuals with TBI, and contributes to increased caregiver strain.

It is now widely recognized that communication problems occurring after TBI are very different from the aphasic disturbances seen following a cerebrovascular accident (CVA) or a more focal injury (Hartley & Griffith, 1989). Much has been written about remediation for aphasia, but this is not the topic in this chapter; the focus is rather on the type of communication difficulties that tend to follow more diffuse injuries, including cognitive communication disorders (CCDs) and social cognition deficits. Ways of building awareness, identifying areas for intervention, developing skills/strategies, and transferring these into everyday situations are considered in this chapter.

THEORETICAL BACKGROUND AND MODELS

Several models and approaches support work on communication difficulties. Some are based at the impairment level, and can be helpful for identifying specific challenges to be targeted in therapy. Others focus on the wider context in which communication takes place; they consider the interaction of various factors, and allow a clinician to hold a broader view of a client and the brain injury's impact on the client. Some models also indicate possible interventions. We focus in this section on models that can be applied more holistically.

Executive Functioning/Cognitive Models

There are many executive functioning/cognitive models which help us to understand communication problems. However, the neuropsychological model for psychological interventions by Grattan and Ghahramanlou (2002) has been useful in bringing together different aspects of brain injury, including the physical injury, its impact on social participation, moderating variables, and suggested interventions.

Social Model of Disability

The social model of disability suggests that disability is not caused by the functional limitations imposed by the impairments a person has, but rather by the failure of society to take account of the person's needs. Social barriers are disabling; these can be environmental, structural, informational, and attitudinal. Byng and Duchan (2006) have developed a framework for therapy for people with aphasia—now adapted to include people with TBI—that is underpinned by the social model of disability.

The framework includes six interrelated goals of therapy (identity, enhancing communication, psychological state, health promotion/illness promotion, access to autonomy and choice, and barriers to social communication) addressed at different levels of social functioning—the immediate social environment, community, and society. Providing therapy within this framework is consistent with a holistic therapeutic approach. We have found the social model of disability especially useful at The Oliver Zangwill Centre, as it allows us to work at an impairment level as well as thinking broadly at a social level (Pound, Parr, Lindsay, & Woolf, 2004).

Framework for Person-Centered, Context-Sensitive Intervention and Support

Mark Ylvisaker and Tim Feeney's framework supports reconstruction of identity after brain injury (Ylvisaker & Feeney, 2000). The model is centered around everyday context-specific routines, with the idea of apprenticeship and collaboration at its heart. Clients are actively involved in meaningful activities with the aim of reconstructing a satisfying sense of self; these include the use of identity maps involving metaphor, as well as self-coaching and project-based interventions. Clients are encouraged to work on goals that are personally meaningful and that directly affect their social participation and sense of self. Gracey, Prince, and Winson explore this topic further in Chapter 9 of this workbook.

NEUROANATOMY OF COMMUNICATION

The neuropathology of communication difficulties is closely linked to the type of injury and location of damage. Language-processing difficulties such as dysphasia and acquired dyslexia, and motor speech disorders such as dyspraxia or dysarthria, usually occur when there has been focal damage (i.e., damage localized to specific areas involved with those abilities). Such damage is more common after CVA, but may occur after TBI as well.

More usually, TBI involves the frontal, temporal, and occipital areas of the brain, and injury is often more diffuse, affecting various abilities linked to these areas (such as executive functioning, attention, speed of processing, memory, and auditory processing). The range of communication difficulties experienced will vary. As noted at the start of this chapter, these difficulties are termed cognitive communication disorders (CCDs).

Social cognition involves processing certain functions in specific areas of the brain (e.g., the inferior frontal gyrus is implicated in emotion recognition, whereas the right temporal area is involved in processing nonverbal information). Depending on the areas of damage, a particular aspect of social cognition may be affected, or multiple difficulties may have a combined impact on social cognition.

COMMON PRESENTING PROBLEMS

Cognitive Communication Disorders

CCDs are impairments of language or communication that are reflective of more generalized cognitive deficits commonly associated with TBI, such as impaired attention, memory, self-monitoring, judgment, and planning (Hagen, 1984). CCDs encompass the following aspects.

Difficulties with Processing Information

Disturbance in information processing can present as difficulty in processing complex oral and written information and inference, alongside intact comprehension of words, phrases, or sentences, or as impaired auditory processing (Royal College of Speech and Language Therapists, 2006). More specific difficulties in this area may include problems with abstract language, verbal reasoning, and auditory processing.

Difficulties with Verbal Expression

Problems with verbal expression can include anomia or word retrieval deficits (e.g., word substitutions, taking longer to access names); difficulties with discourse, such as excessive talkativeness, disorganized/tangential language, imprecise language, or use of socially inappropriate language; and difficulties with conversational discourse/pragmatics, including tangential language, irrelevant conversational responses, and lack of inhibition (Leblanc, De Guise, Feyz, & Lamoureux, 2006).

Deficits in Nonverbal Communication

Problems with nonverbal communication are difficulties in processing nonlinguistic and paralinguistic aspects of language. These aspects include prosody and intonation, as well as behaviors such as posture, eye contact, and facial expression (Freund, Hayter, MacDonald,

Neary, & Wiseman-Hakes, 1994). Clients with CCDs may also have difficulty in comprehending extended oral communications or communications in stressful environments; in reading social cues and adjusting interactive styles to meet situational demands; and in understanding abstract language and verbal reasoning (Leblanc et al., 2006).

Social Cognition Disorders

Deficits in social cognition after brain injury are now more widely recognized (Babbage et al., 2011). These can include difficulties in emotion recognition (i.e., recognizing the feelings, thoughts, and intentions of others and predicting their behavior), as well as problems with managing, regulating, being aware of, and expressing emotions (Grattan & Ghahramanlou, 2002). These kinds of challenges impact upon interpersonal relationships (Wood & Rutterford, 2006) and a person's communicative competence. Social cognition therefore becomes an area of interest in exploring communication challenges.

Social communication difficulties after ABI may be manifestations of underlying cognitive impairments for some people, but sometimes they can be caused by specific difficulties with social cognition. A detailed assessment will identify causal factors. Louise Phillips's framework supports understanding of social cognition impairments and the interaction among three different components, with a view to identifying targeted areas for intervention:

1. *Perception of own emotions:* Individuals' awareness of their own emotions, at a given time or more generally (mood).
2. *Perception of others' emotions:* The ability to recognize and interpret the emotions of others through facial expression, tone of voice, and eye gaze. This includes being able to make inferences, interpret others' communications, and differentiate sarcasm from humor.
3. *Regulation of behavior:* The ways in which individuals adapt their behavior in relation to their perception of their own and others' emotions (e.g., being able to take another person's perspective, showing empathy in relation to another's distress).

ASSESSING COGNITIVE COMMUNICATION AND SOCIAL COGNITION

The interconnection between CCDs and deficits in social cognition needs to be recognized when interventions are being planned, and detailed assessment of these areas is required to ascertain the nature of presenting difficulties. For example, a person presenting with excessive verbal output may have deficits in executive functioning (making self-monitoring difficult) or in social sensitivity (leading to problems in recognizing the thoughts and feelings of others).

Assessment can be a useful way of beginning to develop clients' awareness of their own difficulties. If formal assessments are explained to clients throughout the evaluation process, results can certainly contribute to developing intellectual awareness. Some assessments with good ecological validity—for example, the Functional Assessment of Verbal

Reasoning and Executive Skills (MacDonald & Johnson, 2005)—can imitate real-life tasks and allow clients to relate any struggles they may have in the assessment process to their actual experiences. Questionnaires that explore clients' perceptions of difficulties can also offer valuable insights; the effect is cumulative if a measure is replicated with a client's significant other, as in the La Trobe Communication Questionnaire (Douglas, O'Flaherty, & Snow, 2000). Provided that a sense of safety is maintained, the feedback from the significant other can offer valuable information that can contribute to increasing the individual's awareness of difficulties.

MAKING THE LINKS

As is true for all areas of cognition, behavior, and other functioning, the communication abilities of clients with brain injury are affected by a range of factors. It is important to work with clients to help them understand how their cognitive profiles and emotional responses can have both negative and positive effects on their communication.

For example, listening can be significantly more difficult for those with memory, attention, or executive functioning problems. Clients may find it harder to screen out external distractions when conversing in busy environments, or to hold a topic of conversation in mind over an extended period. Some people with memory difficulties find themselves needing to interrupt during conversations in an attempt to keep track of what is being said. Those with attentional difficulties also sometimes find themselves losing track in a conversation, so they may say something unrelated or fail to respond when they should. Moreover, they may have particular problems in attending to topics or people that they are not very interested in. All of these issues can on occasion lead to conversation breakdown.

Listening abilities can also be affected by anxiety, depression, and irritability, or by physical challenges such as fatigue, hearing problems, or visual impairments. Clients who are anxious may find it difficult to focus their attention in a conversation and may therefore come across as distracted. Similarly, clients who are depressed may not initiate conversations with others readily and may appear to lack interest. Anxiety and lack of confidence can affect someone's ability to engage in conversation altogether.

To keep conversations going successfully, it is likely that clients will need to employ strategies they have developed for other areas in their conversations. It may be harder for those with cognitive challenges to recognize that a conversation is breaking down; furthermore, difficulties with memory, attention, or self-monitoring can all contribute to less balanced conversations.

REHABILITATION: THE EVIDENCE

Cicerone and colleagues (2000) carried out a systematic review of studies to provide evidence and recommendations for cognitive rehabilitation, and to identify the areas that have responded to intervention. Several studies have supported the effectiveness of individualized treatment for cognitive–linguistic deficits after ABI.

In addition, studies by Helffenstein and Wechsler (1982) and Erlich and Sipes (1985) have shown that group intervention focusing on cognitive remediation for functional communication deficits can be effective. Research by Wiseman-Hakes, Stewart, Wasserman, and Schiller (1998) supported the effectiveness of group treatment for improving pragmatic communication skills (social skills) for six subjects with TBI. Group treatment can therefore be successful in addressing different aspects of CCDs.

Cicerone et al. (2000) cited a study (Thomas-Stonell, Johnson, Schuller, & Jutai, 1994) that recommended interventions for specific areas of language impairment—reading comprehension and language formulation—as beneficial. However, several studies have shown benefits in relation to the more general remediation of social and pragmatic communication abilities after TBI. Cicerone et al. (2000) recommend interventions directed at improving pragmatic communication and conversational skills after TBI; addressing these skills in a therapy group has proved to be successful. In situations where this is not possible, providing intervention through conversational partner training with significant others or with support workers may achieve a similar outcome.

EXPLORING COMMUNICATION AND ITS PROBLEMS WITH CLIENTS

Building Awareness

Most clients will have some intellectual awareness of their difficulties at the start of rehabilitation; developing this is always the starting point for communication-focused intervention. In addition to identifying difficulties, it is helpful to find out what strengths remain, as these may be used to compensate for difficulties. In Chapter 1 of this volume, Wilson discusses awareness in more detail.

Video Feedback

Clients' felt experiences in everyday situations lead to the "lightbulb" moments that raise awareness. An important goal in rehabilitation is creating chances for these lightbulb moments to occur. Take any opportunities possible to make videos of clients (with their consent) in a naturalistic conversational setting. Alternatively, preplanned scenarios (e.g., complaining in a restaurant, discussing the weekend with a friend) can be role-played and recorded.

Ask clients to consider what they believe their communication strengths and challenges to be, and to record these on Handout 6.1. (The handout provides an example each of a strength and a challenge.) Try to get the clients to think about what they themselves agree with, rather than what others have told them, and to give examples where possible. Clients can then watch video feedback, either in a group or in a one-to-one setting with you as the therapist, to endorse, elaborate on, or reject the initial reflections. Be clear about what you are asking them to observe; the checklist of communication behaviors provided as Handout 6.2 can help. Having a conversation about something you observed but the client didn't is easier when you have an example to discuss.

Next, revisit clients' initial evaluation of their strengths and challenges: Is there anything they would like to change? For some clients, increasing their awareness of their communication behavior is enough to prompt a change in that behavior. For others, the process of building awareness will allow clearer goals for intervention and therefore clarity about the desired outcomes.

Identifying Areas for Intervention

Once clients have some awareness of their communication strengths and weaknesses, discussions can focus on establishing areas that require intervention to support the attainment of meaningful goals (e.g., to build friendships or establish rapport with others).

Work with clients on identifying the skills required to engage in a conversation successfully. You can use a role-played conversation or a YouTube clip. Important skills include listening; starting, maintaining, ending, and repairing conversations; and turn taking and verbal organization (the structure of verbal expression). Using each client's checklist of strengths and weaknesses, identify areas that support conversation, as well as those that require further development.

DEVELOPING SKILLS AND STRATEGIES

Listening

Discuss why listening is important when we are communicating with others (e.g., to find information, such as directions to get somewhere; to understand, perhaps if someone is obviously angry and we don't know why; for enjoyment, as when listening to music; or to learn, as in a lecture).

Consider why listening may be more challenging after a brain injury, due to difficulties with memory, attention, or executive functioning. Encourage clients to think of examples from their experience. Discuss how mood can affect the ability to listen, sharing examples from your own experience as well as asking clients for theirs. Think about how physical challenges such as pain, hearing/visual impairments, or fatigue can also affect the ability to listen, and talk through some examples.

It may be helpful to describe the different types of listening in which we may engage; these are described below. Discuss with clients everyday examples of each type. Ask them to make notes on examples of the different types of listening they observe during the week.

Competitive/Combative Listening

Competitive or combative listening happens when we are more interested in promoting our own point of view than in understanding or exploring someone else's view. We listen either for openings to take the floor, or for flaws or weak points we can attack. As we pretend to pay attention, we are impatiently waiting for our moment, or internally formulating a rebuttal and planning a devastating comeback that will destroy their argument and make us victorious. This is often seen in political debates.

Passive or Attentive Listening

When we are genuinely interested in hearing and understanding the other person's point of view, we listen attentively and passively. We assume that we hear and understand correctly, but stay passive and do not verify it—for example, when listening to a radio program or a lecture.

Active Listening

Active listening is the single most useful and important listening skill. In active listening, we are also genuinely interested in understanding what the other person is thinking, feeling, or wanting, or what the message means, and we are active in checking out our understanding before we respond with our own new message. We restate or paraphrase our understanding of the other's message and reflect it back to the sender for verification. This verification or feedback process is what makes active listening effective. Examples might be interactions between good friends, or between a client and therapist!

Several strategies can help us become active listeners. Explore these further with clients by watching a clip of a television debate. Identify together the behaviors appearing to show that people are listening (e.g., nodding, clarifying), and those demonstrating that people are not listening (e.g., talking over another person, poor eye contact).

Nonverbal Listening Behaviors

Brainstorm as a group what clients think is meant by "nonverbal behaviors." Aid the discussion by showing a clip of a soap opera with the sound turned down. How can we tell some of what the characters are communicating? Have clients compare their observations with the checklist in Handout 6.3. Some people use more nonverbal behaviors than others. Ask clients to think about family members or friends who use lots of nonverbal behaviors—or who don't use them at all—and to consider how this use, or lack of use, affects interaction.

Next, ask clients to engage in a conversation while trying to use the nonverbal behaviors listed in Handout 6.3. Reflect on how it feels as both a listener and a speaker when these behaviors are used. Make videos of the role plays, and watch the videos with the clients. Encourage clients to reflect on the impact the nonverbal behaviors have.

Verbal Listening Behaviors

With clients, consider the verbal behaviors listed in Handout 6.3, and discuss whether you observed any of these in the video clips or role-plays you watched. In pairs, role-play again, trying to incorporate some of the verbal behaviors alongside the nonverbal behaviors practiced previously. How does it feel as the speaker when the listener uses these behaviors? As the listener, what feels most natural? Sometimes when clients are beginning to use these kinds of communication skills, doing so can feel a bit false! Using a video camera can help clients to see how their use of skills looks to others; it may come across differently from how they might think.

Paraphrasing

Explain to clients that "paraphrasing" means repeating or summarizing what another person has said. Different words can be used, but the meaning must stay the same. Consider this statement:

> "I had a terrible weekend. First, my alarm clock didn't go off, so I started the day behind. I didn't eat breakfast so that I could make my hair appointment at 9:00 A.M. I rushed from there to collect a parcel from the post office, and then to my aunt's house, as she'd had some new furniture delivered and I said I'd help her move it in. Then my cousin arrived and said she had broken up with her boyfriend, so I spent an hour trying to cheer her up. I was due to meet my friends at 5:00 P.M. and had to get home and get changed before I met them, so it was pretty frantic. I got to the restaurant late, and then realized I was in the wrong place, so I rushed to the right restaurant and ended up having a lovely time. However, on Sunday I woke up and realized I had lost my phone, and I spent all day trying to track down where I had left it."

This could be paraphrased as follows: "So you had a pretty hectic weekend, starting with oversleeping, and then having to rush to appointments and deal with family problems. Despite having a nice evening, you found out you had lost your phone." Handout 6.4 offers some practice at paraphrasing.

Clarification

The technique of clarification ensures that we have understood another person's point correctly, and that our understanding and the other person's are the same. The left-hand side of Handout 6.5 offers some examples of clarifying phrases; ask clients to observe other people in conversation to gather more examples. Then role-play conversations using the clarifying phrases, and use video feedback to observe how these phrases help the conversation. Ask clients to consider how it feels when they or others use clarification.

Summarizing

Explain that summarizing involves recapping information in a concise form. Ask clients to read a newspaper article or think of a TV documentary or film they have watched recently. Then ask each client to summarize the article or program to other members of the group. When summarizing, clients may find it helpful to keep in mind the six key questions listed on the right-hand side of Handout 6.5.

Starting Conversations

With clients, make a list of reasons why it might be difficult to initiate a conversation with someone else (e.g., not knowing what to say, worrying that the other person will not understand us, not knowing the other person). Some possible conversation openers are given in

Handout 6.6; brainstorm others with clients. There are certain topics of conversation—"neutral topics"—that are generally inoffensive and so can be used in most situations; consider which of the topics listed in Handout 6.6 could be described as neutral.

Maintaining Conversations

Being able to maintain a conversation successfully with someone presents a challenge to many people, not simply those with brain injury. Problems may include not knowing what to say next to keep a conversation going, difficulties in keeping on topic, problems with linking utterances together, and problems in making a smooth transition from one topic to the next. Many skills are required to keep conversations going. Some people have difficulty in attending to topics or people that they are not very interested in; others find that memory difficulties make it harder to recall what might have previously been said. Anxiety or lack of confidence can also affect someone's ability to engage in conversation.

It is important for clients to be aware of their strengths and weaknesses, and of how other cognitive difficulties may be affecting their communication skills. It is likely that they will need to employ strategies they have developed in other areas in their conversations. The listening strategies identified above can also help maintain conversations.

The left-hand side of Handout 6.7 gives some phrases that can be used to help to keep a conversation going. Ask clients to use these phrases alongside clarifying, paraphrasing, or summarizing in a role-play conversation. Use video feedback and reflection to help the clients consider how this approach feels and comes across.

Repairing Conversations

Repair is used to prevent a breakdown in a conversation or to fix a breakdown that has already occurred. We may need to repair conversations when we have said something unintentionally or if we can see that the other person has misunderstood what we have said. Cognitive challenges can affect clients' ability to recognize that a conversation is breaking down. Discuss with clients any conversations they have had where there was a misunderstanding or the conversations broke down for some reason. What might have contributed to the breakdown? Were there any nonverbal signs that might have suggested the conversations were breaking down? If so, were the clients aware of these? If not, what signs could there have been? At what point in these conversations did the clients realize there was a problem? What did they do? Did they or the other person say anything? How did it feel?

Picking up signs that a conversation is breaking down will offer clues to the best way to repair it. Using some of the strategies described above can help clients to identify difficulties early. For example, paraphrasing or clarifying during a conversation will make it possible to check that both parties are still understanding each other correctly.

Sometimes breakdowns occur with little warning. When this happens, it can lead to awkward silences, embarrassed looks, or even harsh words. In these instances we often say nothing, which can make the situation worse. However, by acknowledging that something has gone wrong and apologizing at the time or soon afterward, we can often quickly remedy the situation. Knowing and being honest about any cognitive challenges can help (e.g., "I'm sorry, I lost my attention for a minute there . . . would you mind going over that last part again?" or "I think I've upset you . . . I'm sorry, I didn't mean to . . . I sometimes get the wrong end of the stick"). Encourage clients to think of one or two stock phrases they will feel comfortable using if they believe an explanation is needed for a conversational breakdown. Ask them to try these phrases out in a role-play situation.

In addition, remind clients that conversations always involve at least one other person, and that a breakdown in conversation is the responsibility of both participants. Ideally, if they identify that something has gone wrong, the other person will help with the repair!

Turn Taking

A balanced conversation requires an element of turn taking. We all know people who talk more than others and may dominate conversations. Equally, there are others who are very quiet in interactions, and the responsibility to keep the conversation going feels as though it's all ours! These differences are often fine and are naturally accepted as part of different people's personalities. However, when a conversation is not balanced, it can cause frustrations and resentment.

Difficulties with memory, attention, or self-monitoring can all contribute to less balanced conversations. Some people with memory difficulties find themselves needing to interrupt during conversations in an effort to remember what's being said. People with attentional difficulties sometimes find themselves losing track in a conversation, so they say something unrelated or don't respond when they should. Difficulties in monitoring may mean that someone talks too much or not enough without realizing it.

Make videos of clients engaged in a discussion or conversation in a group or with someone they know well. Then review the videos and note how long each speaker "has the floor." Are the turns of about equal length among all speakers? Does one speaker speak more than the others? Are there people who are not involved very much in the conversation? Discuss with the group members why it was that one person spoke either more or less. Did cognitive or emotional factors contribute?

The right-hand side of Handout 6.7 lists some ways of getting involved in a conversation when lots of people are talking or another person is talking too much. Make videos of clients engaging in role plays while using some of these strategies, and reflect on the playback.

Some clients may frequently interrupt conversations or talk over others; consider with them why this might be the case. Can they use attention or memory strategies to help them attend to conversations and retain information, avoiding the need for interruptions? Clients might jot down keywords or sketch/doodle something to remind them of points to make later in the conversation; use the mental blackboard or another visual image as a reminder; or use Stop/Think if they are tempted to interrupt. (See the discussions of these and other strategies in Fish & Brentnall, Chapter 4, and Winegardner, Chapter 5, this volume.) Have clients practice the strategies in a group conversation, and encourage the clients to consider which ones work best for them.

Verbal Organization

Some clients may report that conversations may seem confused at times, with jumps from one topic to another. Consider some possible reasons for this. Are the clients assuming that their listeners have more information than they actually do, or are they perhaps giving the listeners too much information? Have they shared personal information without being asked, which can be uncomfortable for listeners? Are the clients' statements specific enough? Or are they perhaps responding to others' questions without actually answering the questions? Again, video feedback can help to raise clients' awareness of difficulties in this area.

Ending Conversations

Being able to end a conversation is just as important as being able to start one! It is important to combine verbal and nonverbal behaviors to get the right message across (e.g., getting up while saying, "Thank you, that was most helpful"). With clients, watch a clip from a soap opera, and focus on how conversations come to an end. How do we know if a person is ending a conversation? Try watching the clip again with the sound turned down; what nonverbal behaviors indicate that a conversation is about to close? Ask clients to consider whether they use any of these. Handout 6.8 lists some verbal and nonverbal cues that can be used to end conversations. Ask clients to use these cues while role-playing the scenarios in the bulleted list at the end of the handout.

Communication Styles

Clients and their families may notice changes in the clients' style of communication after brain injury. Such changes can be subtle, but they may have a significant impact on outcome from rehabilitation, such as return to work and family functioning. It is widely reported that personality changes can be noted after an injury; these may be displayed in communication, but can be difficult for professionals to assess because they have not known the persons before their injury. Using a simple questionnaire such as Handout 6.9 with both a client and a significant other may be helpful in exploring differences between premorbid and postinjury communication styles.

Using Handout 6.10 (which provides words and images in separate boxes that can be cut out), discuss with clients the four common communication behavior types: direct aggression, indirect aggression, assertiveness, and passivity. Ask them to match the adjectives to the different styles.

In order for us to identify different communication styles in ourselves, it is important to recognize them in others. Use clips from YouTube or the video clips provided on The Oliver Zangwill Centre's website (*www.ozc.nhs.uk*) to identify the different behavior types seen. Turn down the sound and focus on the nonverbal communication observed; consider posture, eye contact, gesture, proximity, and facial expression. Then, with the sound turned up, ask clients to think about aspects of verbal communication such as tone of voice, speech volume, and speed of speech.

Next, ask the group to carry out the role plays listed below, taking on different roles and behavior styles. Discuss beforehand what verbal and nonverbal behaviors would be appropriate for each style. Make videos of the role plays and review these, remembering that feedback from peers within a group can be very powerful. (You can also encourage clients to discuss real-life experiences they have had.)

- It is late at night, and your neighbor is playing loud music for the third night in a row. You go next door to ask him to turn it down.
- The TV repair person was supposed to come to your house at 10:00 A.M. It is now 1:00 P.M., and you have to go to work, having already taken the morning off. You call the shop to complain.
- You need to take time off work to attend your daughter's graduation, but you know your boss has a big job needing to be completed. You arrange an appointment with him to talk about it.
- You have lent a friend some money, but 2 weeks have passed and he has not repaid it.
- A colleague at work asked you out on a date; you reluctantly agreed, but you wish you had not and want to back out.

Although there is no right or wrong communication style, it is important to be aware of the effects our communication styles might have on others and ourselves. Discuss the effects of the different styles. Ask how clients felt both when they were being assertive, directly aggressive, indirectly aggressive, or passive, and when they were on the receiving end of these behaviors. For example, direct aggression may give feelings of power or act as a way of releasing tension, or it can lead to feelings of guilt or shame as a person displaces responsibility for his or her anger. The ultimate consequence of this guilt or shame can be loss of self-confidence and self-esteem or resentment in others. Indirect aggression is harder to pin down, as it is more subtle than direct aggression. It creates an undercurrent of guilty unease in the listener, but may in the short term boost the speaker's self-esteem as he or she manipulates the listener and avoids direct expression of feelings. Short-term effects of passive behaviors can include reduction or avoidance of guilt and a sense of martyrdom; over a longer period, passive behaviors can create increased internal tensions, leading to stress, anger, depression, and loss of self-esteem.

An assertive approach can be helpful for both ourselves and others. Being open and direct, respecting our own and others' rights, and confidently expressing both positive and negative feelings and opinions can result in improved self-confidence and mutual respect. Assertiveness also involves the ability to take responsibility for ourselves and our actions without judging or blaming other people, and to find compromise where conflict exists.

It is widely felt that in order to develop assertive behaviors, we need to have some underlying beliefs. Holland and Ward (1990) define this set of beliefs as the "Rights Charter," and you may wish to explore this further with clients. Holland and Ward also suggest certain "tools" that help us to develop an assertive behavior style.

Body Language

Discuss what body language might be associated with assertive behavior. Ask clients to act out some scenarios, using different postures and nonverbal behaviors. Encourage them to identify which ones give them a feeling or appearance of confidence.

Setting the Scene

Considering the circumstances in which a difficult conversation takes place can be helpful. These circumstances may include a client's own and the other person's mood, the timing, the setting, and who else is around. Encourage clients to focus on stating how they are feeling, rather than on blaming or criticizing the other person, and to use phrases like "I feel . . ." or "I need . . .". Remind them also to talk about the behavior rather than the person; to be concise and specific; and to stick to their guns while acknowledging the other person's position and respecting his or her rights.

The Broken Record

The "echo technique" is a useful method that can work in virtually any situation. Clients rehearse stating clearly what they want or need, and returning to these prepared lines throughout the conversation.

Scripts

Helping clients to plan what they want to say in a structured way in advance can also be useful. Here are four sets of factors for clients to consider in preparing a "script":

1. The event: The situation, relationship, or practical problem that is important to them.
2. Their feelings: How they feel about the situation, relationship, or problem.
3. Their needs: What they want to happen to make things different.
4. The consequences: How making these positive changes will improve the situation for them and/or others.

It is important to bear in mind that being assertive requires compromise; it is not winning at all costs. The aim should be to avoid a stalemate, and instead to reach a mutual agreement or solution that satisfies both parties.

The best way of developing all these skills is practice. Spend time discussing, planning, and role-playing both imaginary and real-life scenarios; perhaps a problem a client is currently facing can be used. Make videos, review these, and reflect on how the outcome feels for both the speaker and the listener in each video.

BRINGING IT ALL TOGETHER

The next step in the rehabilitation of communication deficits is to transfer strategies developed for overcoming specific difficulties into relevant everyday situations. Transferring and then generalizing strategies may not necessarily happen automatically, and clients can benefit from clinician-led processes as they work toward these goals.

One way of achieving transfer and generalization is by using a project-based approach (Ylvisaker, 2003). Projects are extremely useful in facilitating generalization of strategies, as the main focus tends to be on achieving something that is meaningful to the clients, while the clinician stands alongside and coaches each client to use the relevant strategies where needed. The key ingredient is identifying what is meaningful to each client, as this will motivate the client to use the strategies. Projects can be carried out within a group or individually, depending on the resources available. They require a little thought, planning, and creativity, but, if devised in collaboration with clients, they offer great opportunities for the clients to safely begin generalizing strategies learned in therapy to everyday life. Some projects that have been successfully completed with clients in the past are discussed by Gracey et al. in Chapter 9 of this volume.

Other clients may find that they need more context-specific activities in order to generalize strategies, such as making phone calls to inquire about bank accounts, ordering food in restaurants, or making complaints in stores. Behavioral experiments are useful ways of building confidence in relation to communication skills, and they allow for the introduction of strategies in a situation that is planned to some extent, thereby reducing some of the anxiety. A graded hierarchy or goal ladder can be devised to push clients gently further as their confidence develops. More details about behavioral experiments are given by Winegardner in Chapter 5 and by Ford in Chapter 8 of this volume.

Whether a project-based or a context-specific approach is adopted, it is vital to work with clients and their significant others to identify tasks or activities that are personally meaningful to the clients. These types of tasks will have a greater influence on clients' generalization of strategies and will increase their confidence in their developing skills.

CASE STUDY

The case of Jeff, whose severe TBI in a traffic accident at age 19 cut short his plans for accepting a golf scholarship in the United States, has been introduced by Fish and colleagues at the end of Chapter 3. The problems Jeff faced with regard to communication, and some of his goals and strategies for dealing with these problems, are described in Table 6.1.

TABLE 6.1. Dealing with Jeff's Communication Challenges

Challenges	Goals and strategies	Context for rehabilitation
Limited range of conversation topics and poor topic control Jeff could talk at length about golf, but found it difficult to switch topics or take into account his conversation partner's interests. *Poor initiation and maintenance of conversations* Jeff tended not to initiate or ask questions. He often gave one-word answers without elaboration; as a result, his conversations often fizzled out quickly. *Poor awareness of communication style* Jeff lacked insight into his communication difficulties. He was also unaware that people sometimes had difficulty understanding him because he spoke very rapidly at times, especially when he was anxious. *Occasionally impulsive and socially inappropriate behavior* Jeff had made some suggestive remarks to a female member of his golf club, resulting in a complaint against him.	Goal: To improve communication skills with a view to starting a relationship. Techniques for building awareness: • Video feedback • Psychoeducation • Monitoring and feedback from staff and peers	Jeff was keen to try speed dating; therapy sessions focused on building up to this goal. Video feedback from Jeff's communication in other contexts was reviewed, to build his awareness of his difficulties and his sense of what is and isn't socially appropriate. A one-to-one practice session was held in the first instance, with feedback from the therapist. The GMF (see Winegardner, Chapter 5, this volume) was used to help Jeff decide what to wear and think of a broad range of conversational topics. Jeff practiced slowing down his speech when chairing community meetings and delivering news items. Staff members gave feedback on his performance. When Jeff felt confident enough, a mock speed-dating session was held in the center. He had 3-minute "dates," with six staff members playing various roles, and received positive feedback afterward. Finally, Jeff was supported to investigate real-life speed-dating opportunities in his local area.

REFERENCES

Babbage, D. R., Yim, J., Zupan, B., Newman, D., Tomita, M. R., & Willer, B. (2011). Meta-analysis of facial affect recognition difficulties after Traumatic Brain Injury. *Neuropsychology, 25*(3), 277–285.

Byng, S., & Duchan, J. (2006). A framework for describing therapies and discovering their whys and wherefores. In S. Byng, J. Duchan, & C. Pound (Eds.), *The aphasia therapy file* (Vol. 2, pp. 231–277). Hove, UK: Psychology Press.

Cicerone, K. D., Dahlberg, C., Kalmar, K., Langenbahn, D. M., Malec, J. F., Bergquist, T. F., . . . Morse, P. A. (2000). Evidence-based cognitive rehabilitation: Recommendations for clinical practice. *Archives of Physical Medicine and Rehabilitation, 81*, 1596–1615.

Douglas, J., O'Flaherty, C. A., & Snow, P. C. (2000). Measuring perception of communicative ability: The development and evaluation of the La Trobe Communication Questionnaire. *Aphasiology, 14*(3), 251–268.

Erlich, J., & Sipes, A. (1985). Group treatment of communication skills for head trauma patients. *Cognitive Rehabilitation, 3*, 32–37.

Freund, J., Hayter, C., MacDonald, S., Neary, M. A., & Wiseman-Hakes, C. (1994). *Cognitive communication disorders following traumatic brain injury: A practical guide.* Tucson, AZ: Communication Skill Builders.

Grattan, L., & Ghahramanlou, M. (2002). The rehabilitation of neurologically based social disturbances. In P. Eslinger (Ed.), *Neuropsychological interventions: Clinical research and practice* (pp. 266–293). New York: Guilford Press.

Hagen, C. (1984). Language disorders in head trauma. In A. Holland (Ed.), *Language disorders in adults: Recent advances* (pp. 245–281). San Diego, CA: College Hill Press.

Hartley, L., & Griffith, A. (1989). A functional approach to the cognitive-communication difficulties of closed head injured clients. *Journal of Speech–Language Pathology and Audiology, 13*(2), 51–56.

Helffenstein, D., & Wechsler, R. (1982). The use of interpersonal process recall (IPR) in the remediation of interpersonal and communication skill deficits in the newly brain injured. *Clinical Neuropsychology, 4,* 139–143.

Holland, S., & Ward, C. (1990). *Assertiveness: A practical approach.* Chesterfield, UK: Winslow Press.

Leblanc, J., De Guise, E., Feyz, M., & Lamoureux, J. (2006). Early prediction of language impairment following traumatic brain injury. *Brain Injury, 20*(13–14), 1391–1401.

MacDonald, S., & Johnson, C. J. (2005). Assessment of subtle cognitive communication deficits following acquired brain injury: A normative study of the Functional Assessment of Verbal Reasoning and Executive Strategies. *Brain Injury, 19*(11), 895–902.

Pound, C., Parr, S., Lindsay, J., & Woolf, C. (2004). *Beyond aphasia: Therapies for living with communication disability.* Oxford, UK: Speechmark.

Royal College of Speech and Language Therapists. (2006). *Communicating quality 3.* London: Author.

Struchen, M. A., Clark, A. N., Sander, A. M., Mills, M. R., Evans, G., & Kurtz, D. (2008). Relation of executive functioning and social communication measures to functional outcomes following traumatic brain injury. *NeuroRehabilitation, 23,* 185–198.

Thomas-Stonell, N., Johnson, P., Schuller, R., & Jutai, J. (1994). Evaluation of a computer based program for cognitive-communication skills. *Journal of Head Trauma Rehabilitation, 9*(4), 25–37.

Wiseman-Hakes, C., Stewart, M. L., Wasserman, R., & Schiller, R. (1998). Peer group training of pragmatic skills in adolescents with acquired brain injury. *Journal of Head Trauma Rehabilitation, 13*(6), 23–38.

Wood, R., & Rutterford, N. (2006). Demographic and cognitive predictors of long-term psychosocial outcome following traumatic brain injury. *Journal of the International Neuropsychological Society, 12*(3), 350–358.

Ylvisaker, M. (2003). Context-sensitive cognitive rehabilitation after brain injury: Theory and practice. *Brain Impairment, 4*(1), 1–16.

Ylvisaker, M., & Feeney, T. J. (2000). Construction of identity after traumatic brain injury. *Brain Impairment, 1,* 12–28.

Communication Skills: Strengths and Challenges

Strengths	Challenges
Example: Good listener	*Example: Keeping up in groups*

From *The Brain Injury Rehabilitation Workbook*, edited by Rachel Winson, Barbara A. Wilson, and Andrew Bateman. Copyright © 2017 The Guilford Press. Permission to photocopy this handout is granted to purchasers of this book for personal use or for use with individual clients (see copyright page for details). Purchasers can download additional copies of this handout (see the box at the end of the table of contents).

Communication Behaviors Checklist

Place a check mark next to any of the following behaviors you observe during the conversation. Make a brief note of what you saw.

☐ Eye contact

☐ Body language

☐ Facial expression

☐ Listening

☐ Distance between speakers

☐ Tone of voice

☐ Volume of voice

☐ Getting the point across

From *The Brain Injury Rehabilitation Workbook*, edited by Rachel Winson, Barbara A. Wilson, and Andrew Bateman. Copyright © 2017 The Guilford Press. Permission to photocopy this handout is granted to purchasers of this book for personal use or for use with individual clients (see copyright page for details). Purchasers can download additional copies of this handout (see the box at the end of the table of contents).

Communication Behaviors Observations Sheet

Nonverbal Listening Behaviors

Facial expressions: Angry, surprised, sad, disgusted, worried, happy

Use of gestures: Finger pointing, finger shaking, fist waving, using hands for emphasis

Head/body movements: Nodding, shaking head, head down, shoulders hunched, shoulders straight, open posture

Proximity: Standing close to someone, moving away from someone

Verbal Listening Behaviors

"Uh-huh."

"Yes."

"Hmmm."

"Right."

"Oh."

"Really?"

"Gosh!"

"I see."

"OK."

"Really!"

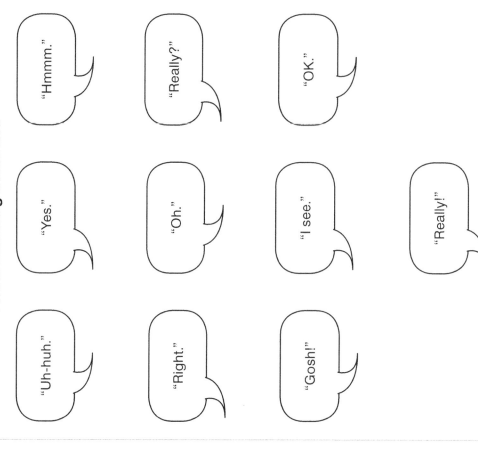

From *The Brain Injury Rehabilitation Workbook*, edited by Rachel Winson, Barbara A. Wilson, and Andrew Bateman. Copyright © 2017 The Guilford Press. Permission to photocopy this handout is granted to purchasers of this book for personal use or for use with individual clients (see copyright page for details). Purchasers can download additional copies of this handout (see the box at the end of the table of contents).

Paraphrasing

Paraphrase the following statements.

1. "Today I was running really late for work, and then my car wouldn't start. I finally got it going— but, as you know, the roads were really icy this morning, so then I skidded halfway down the street. If that wasn't enough, the fuel gauge light came on, so I only had just enough in the tank to get me here. I'll have to fill up the car after work."

_____

_____

_____

_____

_____

_____

2. "On Saturday I took the girls shopping, as they both needed new shoes. We decided to have a snack in town, and then we went to the park—you know, the one with the big pirate ship—before having ice cream on the way home."

_____

_____

_____

_____

_____

_____

3. "This morning was typical for a Monday. There must have been a blackout during the night, or somehow we lost power, because my alarm didn't go off and I managed to oversleep. But, fortunately, I was ready in time for my ride to work."

_____

_____

_____

_____

_____

_____

From *The Brain Injury Rehabilitation Workbook*, edited by Rachel Winson, Barbara A. Wilson, and Andrew Bateman. Copyright © 2017 The Guilford Press. Permission to photocopy this handout is granted to purchasers of this book for personal use or for use with individual clients (see copyright page for details). Purchasers can download additional copies of this handout (see the box at the end of the table of contents).

Clarifying and Summarizing

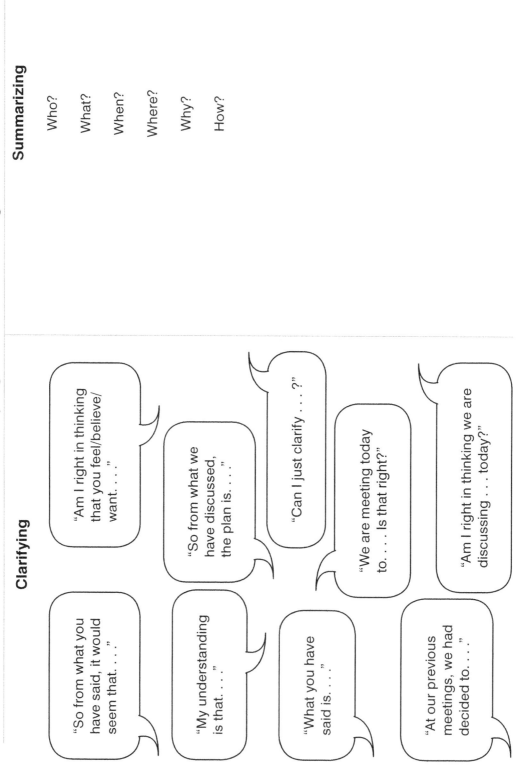

Clarifying

"So from what you have said, it would seem that. . . ."

"Am I right in thinking that you feel/believe/want. . . ."

"My understanding is that. . . ."

"So from what we have discussed, the plan is. . . ."

"What you have said is. . . ."

"Can I just clarify . . . ?"

"At our previous meetings, we had decided to. . . ."

"We are meeting today to. . . . Is that right?"

"Am I right in thinking we are discussing . . . today?"

Summarizing

Who?

What?

When?

Where?

Why?

How?

From *The Brain Injury Rehabilitation Workbook*, edited by Rachel Winson, Barbara A. Wilson, and Andrew Bateman. Copyright © 2017 The Guilford Press. Permission to photocopy this handout is granted to purchasers of this book for personal use or for use with individual clients (see copyright page for details). Purchasers can download additional copies of this handout (see the box at the end of the table of contents).

Starting Conversations

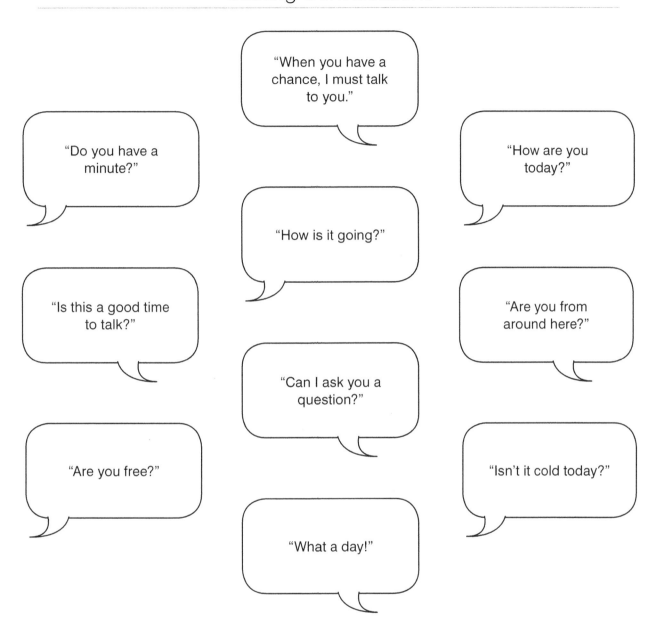

"When you have a chance, I must talk to you."

"Do you have a minute?"

"How are you today?"

"How is it going?"

"Is this a good time to talk?"

"Are you from around here?"

"Can I ask you a question?"

"Are you free?"

"Isn't it cold today?"

"What a day!"

Which of these topics are OK for starting a conversation? Which are hot topics best avoided?

Holidays	Your children	Your health issues
Weather	Religion	Politics

Comments on your surroundings

From *The Brain Injury Rehabilitation Workbook*, edited by Rachel Winson, Barbara A. Wilson, and Andrew Bateman. Copyright © 2017 The Guilford Press. Permission to photocopy this handout is granted to purchasers of this book for personal use or for use with individual clients (see copyright page for details). Purchasers can download additional copies of this handout (see the box at the end of the table of contents).

Maintaining Conversations and Taking Turns

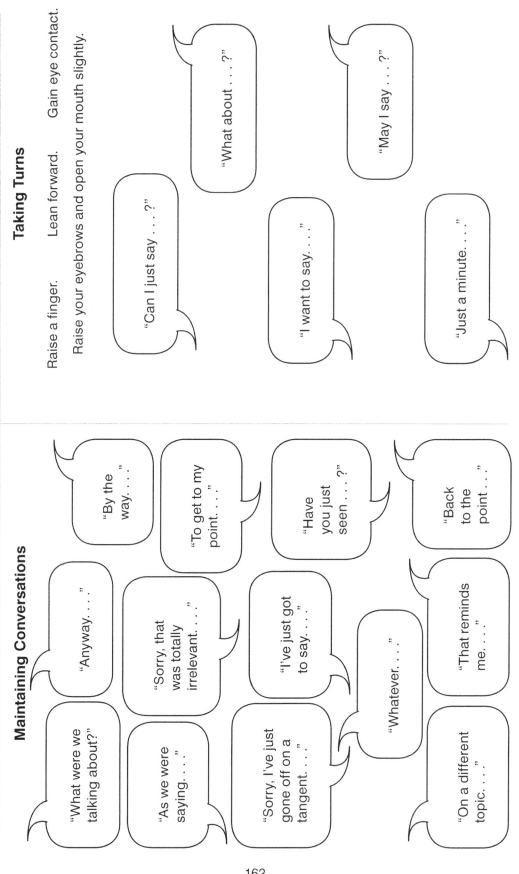

Taking Turns

Raise a finger. Lean forward. Gain eye contact.

Raise your eyebrows and open your mouth slightly.

"Can I just say . . . ?"

"What about . . . ?"

"I want to say. . . ."

"May I say . . . ?"

"Just a minute. . . ."

Maintaining Conversations

"By the way. . . ."

"To get to my point. . . ."

"Have you just seen . . . ?"

"Back to the point. . . ."

"Anyway. . . ."

"Sorry, that was totally irrelevant. . . ."

"I've just got to say. . . ."

"Whatever. . . ."

"That reminds me. . . ."

"What were we talking about?"

"As we were saying. . . ."

"Sorry, I've just gone off on a tangent. . . ."

"On a different topic. . . ."

From *The Brain Injury Rehabilitation Workbook*, edited by Rachel Winson, Barbara A. Wilson, and Andrew Bateman. Copyright © 2017 The Guilford Press. Permission to photocopy this handout is granted to purchasers of this book for personal use or for use with individual clients (see copyright page for details). Purchasers can download additional copies of this handout (see the box at the end of the table of contents).

Ending Conversations

Nonverbal Cues

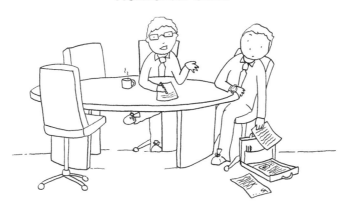

Turning away   Standing up   Looking down   Looking at the clock

Packing things up around you   Opening the door

Looking at other people

Verbal Cues

"I'm really sorry, but I have to go now."

"It's been really interesting talking to you."

"OK, I think we've covered everything."

"So can we set up another time to meet?"

"Good to meet you. See you again."

"I just need to catch someone else . . . please excuse me."

Role-play the following situations, using some of the nonverbal and verbal cues listed above.

- You are in a rush and can't talk.
- The topic makes you feel uncomfortable.
- You are bored or not interested.
- Someone else catches your eye.

From *The Brain Injury Rehabilitation Workbook*, edited by Rachel Winson, Barbara A. Wilson, and Andrew Bateman. Copyright © 2017 The Guilford Press. Permission to photocopy this handout is granted to purchasers of this book for personal use or for use with individual clients (see copyright page for details). Purchasers can download additional copies of this handout (see the box at the end of the table of contents).

Social Communication Skills Questionnaire

Observation	Do you notice this?	Is this a change since your injury?	Example
1. Difficulties demonstrating or communicating feelings.	Yes No	Yes No	
2. Being overemotional or unemotional.	Yes No	Yes No	
3. Difficulties with judging when is an appropriate time (or place) to talk about particular topics.	Yes No	Yes No	
4. Difficulties with choosing a topic of conversation (or question) in keeping with the social situation.	Yes No	Yes No	
5. Tendency to dominate conversations or to withdraw completely from conversations.	Yes No	Yes No	
6. Standing or sitting too close to others.	Yes No	Yes No	
7. Too much/too little eye contact.	Yes No	Yes No	
8. Too much/not enough touching with some people.	Yes No	Yes No	
9. Difficulty with interpreting other people's facial expressions.	Yes No	Yes No	
10. Facial expression that doesn't match what is said.	Yes No	Yes No	
11. Difficulties in understanding jokes.	Yes No	Yes No	

(continued)

From *The Brain Injury Rehabilitation Workbook*, edited by Rachel Winson, Barbara A. Wilson, and Andrew Bateman. Copyright © 2017 The Guilford Press. Permission to photocopy this handout is granted to purchasers of this book for personal use or for use with individual clients (see copyright page for details). Purchasers can download additional copies of this handout (see the box at the end of the table of contents).

Observation	Do you notice this?	Is this a change since your injury?	Example
12. Problems with putting yourself "in someone else's shoes" and changing your behavior to accommodate this.	Yes No	Yes No	
13. Difficulties with being sympathetic to others in distress.	Yes No	Yes No	
14. Being too apologetic or too complimentary to others.	Yes No	Yes No	
15. Any other examples of changes in social interaction or emotional processing?			

Communication Styles

Bossy	Sarcastic
Bulldozing	Insinuating
Arrogant	Devious
Overbearing	Manipulative
Opinionated	Guilt-inducing
Intolerant	Ambiguous
Direct	Waiting
Honest	Moaning
Positive	Helpless
Spontaneous	Submissive
Accepting	Indecisive
Responsible	Apologetic

From *The Brain Injury Rehabilitation Workbook*, edited by Rachel Winson, Barbara A. Wilson, and Andrew Bateman. Copyright © 2017 The Guilford Press. Permission to photocopy this handout is granted to purchasers of this book for personal use or for use with individual clients (see copyright page for details). Purchasers can download additional copies of this handout (see the box at the end of the table of contents).

CHAPTER 7

Fatigue

Donna Malley

Fatigue is one of the most commonly reported symptoms after acquired brain injury (ABI), with an estimated incidence of over 60% across the range of injury severity following traumatic brain injury (TBI) (Ponsford et al., 2012). It may occur in the acute and postacute stages after onset of ABI, and for some clients it may persist over time. Understanding, defining, and assessing fatigue are challenging, as many confounding factors are associated with it. "Pathological fatigue," which warrants clinical attention, is defined as fatigue that does not dissipate with rest and is of greater intensity and duration than "normal fatigue" following exertion. It significantly reduces an individual's ability to participate in rehabilitation and daily living activities. Chronic fatigue has a negative impact on mood, identity, relationships, and quality of life, and those who experience it describe it as qualitatively different from the type of fatigue they experienced prior to their brain injury.

It is important to acknowledge and understand the personal experience and impact of fatigue on each individual following brain injury. Experience of chronic fatigue can influence a person's sense of identity, in part because the person is unable to participate fully in the desired roles and activities that help to define him or her. The timing, content, and process of fatigue management need to be individualized; a linear approach to assessment and intervention is not always possible or appropriate, particularly if psychosocial variables are major contributing factors. Both psychoeducational group sessions and individual intervention, delivered by a multiprofessional team, are likely to optimize fatigue management.

This chapter provides the following:

- Information for clinicians about fatigue following brain injury: theoretical and practical considerations for assessment, intervention, and evaluation.
- Handouts and activity suggestions to help clients understand why they experience fatigue.
- Suggestions for management strategies to help clients make the best use of their available resources.

THEORETICAL BACKGROUND AND MODELS

Fatigue is now widely accepted as a multidimensional, biopsychosocial construct, with physiological and psychological factors influencing its presentation and felt experience within societal and cultural contexts. Several models of fatigue have been proposed in the literature, including fatigue associated with neurological conditions in general (Kluger, Krupp, & Enoka, 2013) and stroke in particular (Eilertsen, Ormstad, & Kirkevold, 2013; Lerdal et al., 2009; Wu, Mead, Macleod, & Chalder, 2015). However, these models have not been found to be clinically useful, and so a clinical model of persistent fatigue following ABI, based on a synthesis of evidence and clinical practice, has been developed to guide assessment and intervention (Malley, Wheatcroft, & Gracey, 2014). Use of this model can facilitate a shared understanding between individuals who experience persistent fatigue following ABI and their caregivers/families. It also provides a rationale for further assessment and intervention. Figure 7.1 presents a schematic diagram of the model for reference here, and Handout 7.1 presents it in a form that can be shared with clients and others.*

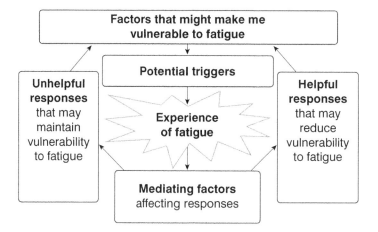

FIGURE 7.1. Model of fatigue following acquired brain injury (ABI).

---

*All handouts are at the end of the chapter.

The model suggests that fatigue is influenced by predisposing or vulnerability factors, which may include previous life experiences and comorbid illness, alongside injury-related primary and secondary fatigue factors. The primary and secondary factors that could be contributing to fatigue are determined through assessment of pathology, physiology, and associated physical, cognitive, and psychosocial factors. Potential triggers (activities or situations), the felt experience of fatigue (including thoughts, feelings, sensations, and behaviors), and mediating factors that influence how an individual responds (either to perpetuate the fatigue or to ameliorate the experience) can then be identified. This model can be used with clients to create a shared understanding or formulation of the mechanisms involved in their fatigue following ABI, and thereby to support identification of factors influencing coping responses to facilitate appropriate intervention.

In the planning of fatigue management, it may be possible to address both primary and/or secondary causes and consequences of fatigue. The vulnerability factors and triggers influencing fatigue need to be considered alongside the mediating factors in order to consider how an individual may respond to various management strategies, and to support the individual in developing such strategies. The clinical goals of fatigue management are thus to create a shared understanding of each client's experience of and responses to fatigue, increase the individual's ability to participate in desired activities, develop personalized management strategies, and reduce the psychological distress associated with fatigue.

The remainder of this chapter is based upon this clinical model.

NEUROANATOMY OF FATIGUE

Many people experience profound tiredness or lack of energy following brain injury, but the underlying causes and taxonomy remain poorly understood and much debated. "Peripheral fatigue" is defined as a diminished ability to contract muscles, involving the peripheral motor and sensory systems (Elovic, Dobrovic, & Fellus, 2005), and may result from injuries sustained alongside TBI; however, the focus of this chapter is on "central fatigue" or "primary fatigue," which is associated with disruption to the central nervous system. This type of fatigue may be a result of mechanical damage to brain structures (e.g., the hypothalamus, leading to hypopituitarism) and connections (e.g., the ascending reticular activating system), or it may result from impaired excitability of the motor cortex. Fatigue may also occur as a secondary consequence of other factors associated with ABI, such as poor sleep, pain, mood disorders, and cognitive dysfunction; this type of fatigue is known as "secondary fatigue." Ponsford and colleagues (2012) provide a good summary of the mechanisms involved in fatigue associated with TBI, whereas Duncan, Wu, and Mead (2012) and Crosby, Munshi, Karat, Worthington, and Lincoln (2012) discuss fatigue associated with stroke. Clinically, fatigue associated with ABI is likely to include all of these aspects. One of a clinician's roles is to consider these different factors and their interactions in determining personal vulnerability factors.

MAKING THE LINKS

As indicated earlier, secondary fatigue is considered to be associated with exertion involved in managing other consequences of the brain injury—physical, cognitive, emotional, and social—as a person interacts with his or her environment. Evidence suggests that reduced speed of processing and attention difficulties are associated with mental fatigue (Ponsford et al., 2012). Fatigue can be a symptom of depression, although it can also occur independently of it. Coping styles and difficulty adjusting to an injury can also contribute to fatigue. Secondary fatigue is most likely to occur as an interaction among these factors, physiological changes, and the activities a client wants and needs to do. Sometimes vicious cycles can result, in which a person tries to do something, struggles to think and makes errors, feels fatigued from the effort, and then feels critical of his or her own efforts; the person then avoids the activity and feels low in mood, and the avoidance and low mood exacerbate the fatigue. This is one of the reasons why it is so tricky to work out how best to manage an individual's fatigue, and why several different strategies used together are likely to work best.

Fatigue can also be a consequence of either a preexisting or new medical condition, and/or a side effect of certain types of medication. It is therefore important to seek advice from a medical professional to rule out other possible causes of fatigue. Other medical conditions that may contribute to fatigue following a brain injury include hormone deficiencies (e.g., hypopituitarism), vitamin D deficiency, sleep disorders, anemia, or a need for frequent urination (which can disrupt sleep). Sometimes side effects of medication may include drowsiness, which contributes further toward a person's feeling tired during the day. It is therefore important to discuss possible side effects of medication, and to consider possible alternatives that have fewer side effects. However, the person should be advised not to stop taking any medications or to change any dosages without discussing this first with his or her general practitioner (GP) or primary care provider (PCP), or with a medication consultant.

Medication may be helpful in managing other factors associated with brain injury. For example, antidepressants for low mood, or hormone replacements in cases of hormone deficiency, can significantly reduce the fatigue that people experience. However, there is currently very little evidence to support a direct effect of medication on fatigue following brain injury. Some types of medication have been found to be helpful in other conditions where fatigue is a symptom (e.g., modafinil for people who experience excessive daytime sleepiness).

COMMON PRESENTING PROBLEMS

The experience of fatigue following brain injury is very different from that of fatigue before the injury occurred. Individuals report that it can feel out of proportion to what they have been doing. It may come over them unexpectedly and last for some time, even after resting. Other people may not understand this, which can cause difficulties with interpersonal relationships and contribute to misunderstandings between clients and these others. Clients describe this kind of fatigue as overwhelming and unpleasant, and report that it sometimes feels out of their control. Handout 7.2 offers some quotes from clients and a visual depiction of how fatigue can feel.

Fatigue can affect what people think, how they feel, and what they do. For some, the tiredness may feel so overwhelming that they are unable to complete normal activities of daily living. People may say that they feel exhausted, lacking in energy, weak, or very sleepy; that they have difficulty motivating themselves; or that the fatigue is accompanied by headaches or aching limbs. For others, fatigue may exacerbate difficulties associated with their brain injury (e.g., forgetfulness, irritability, slurred speech, distractibility, dizziness). Because fatigue often makes planning ahead or resuming previous roles and daily activities more difficult, it can have a major impact on a person's sense of self.

Those who experience persistent fatigue after brain injury describe three types:

- "Physical fatigue" is described as occurring when limbs feel heavy, muscles ache, or people feel clumsy. It usually occurs after a period of physical exertion or exercise. Many people don't find this type of fatigue unpleasant or worrying, but accept it as a natural part of their condition and recovery, and as an understandable consequence of doing activities.

- "Mental fatigue" is fatigue that affects the ability to think. Therapists may refer to this as "cognitive fatigue." It is harder to concentrate, remember information, make decisions, solve problems, and initiate doing things; as a result of all these difficulties, people often make errors, which then have a negative impact on their feelings about themselves. This type of fatigue may be confusing and is often misunderstood by others. Sometimes people may feel that the thinking involved in an activity doesn't warrant the mental fatigue they experience, and this belief too can be very frustrating and can affect how they respond.

- "Emotional fatigue" may affect not only feelings, but thoughts and behaviors. Constant worrying (ruminating) uses energy and can contribute toward clients' feeling more emotional, more tearful, more irritable, or angrier. These feelings can then influence how they communicate with and behave toward other people, and how other people react toward them. This type of fatigue is confusing, may be difficult to describe, and therefore may easily be misunderstood.

Following brain injury, people may need increased time and have to make more mental effort to think and perform tasks. Many people experience difficulty sustaining this effort over time. Some people have described reaching a point at which their brains just "shut off": for example, "It's just like this cloud that comes over . . . my brain will shut off, it just can't cope with it . . . I feel I need to shut down." In addition, cognitive difficulties that are direct results of the brain injury may be exacerbated by fatigue. Making the best use of remaining cognitive resources through applying well-learned compensatory strategies may be a way not only to maximize clients' abilities, but to decrease their fatigue. Effort and energy will be required to learn new ways of coping, and clients may need to be supported to practice these new ways until they become habits. Once these habits are formed, however, they should reduce the effort clients need to make, and also increase the likelihood of successful outcomes.

ASSESSING FATIGUE AND ITS IMPACT

There is currently no consistently used, clinically valid, and reliable measure for fatigue following ABI. Available fatigue scales, many of which have been developed for different clinical populations, may address different aspects of fatigue. For example, Ponsford and colleagues (2012) recommend using the Fatigue Severity Scale (Krupp, La Rocca, Muir-Nash, & Steinberg, 1989) after TBI to assess the impact of fatigue on daily activities. Other measures typically used by brain injury rehabilitation teams (e.g., the Profile of Mood States; Elbers et al., 2012) may have fatigue subscales.

It is important to keep in mind that objective fatigue and subjective fatigue may not correlate with each other. Feedback from some people with fatigue who experience neuropsychological difficulties following ABI indicates that many fatigue scales do not capture their subjective experience, and some clients have even reported psychological reactions as a consequence of responding to specific questionnaires. Therefore, the choice of measures for assessing fatigue and of associated measures needs to be made with each client's clinical questions and goals for intervention in mind.

Self-report of persistent fatigue following ABI—fatigue that is having a negative impact on psychological well-being and participation in daily living activities—warrants clinical consideration. The assessment process (see Figure 7.2) should incorporate clinical review of all factors outlined in the model described above.

EVALUATION OF OUTCOMES

The desired outcomes of fatigue management may differ for each client and are probably best captured through individual client goal setting. Handout 7.3 offers a questionnaire for evaluating the processes involved in fatigue management alongside achievement of functional goals.

REHABILITATION: THE EVIDENCE

Despite the abundant evidence that persistent fatigue is frequently reported after brain injury and has a major impact on quality of life, evidence to guide clinical interventions for it remains inadequate (Kutlubaev, Mead, & Lerdal, 2015; Cantor et al., 2014; Ponsford & Sinclair, 2014; Ponsford et al., 2012). Survivors of brain injury report a lack of understanding and attention to this symptom by clinicians, caregivers, and family members alike. As indicated previously, what evidence there is suggests that a number of interacting biopsychosocial factors may be associated with a person's experience of and responses to fatigue following ABI. These include sleep disturbance (Ponsford & Sinclair, 2014; Schnieders, Willemsen, & De Boer, 2012); pain (Miller et al., 2013; Crosby et al., 2012; Hoang et al., 2012); cognitive impairments, such as slowed speed of processing, difficulty sustaining attention, and executive dysfunction (Radman et al., 2012; Ronnback & Johansson, 2012; Ponsford et al., 2012); and psychological factors, such as reward and effort perception (Pardini, Krueger,

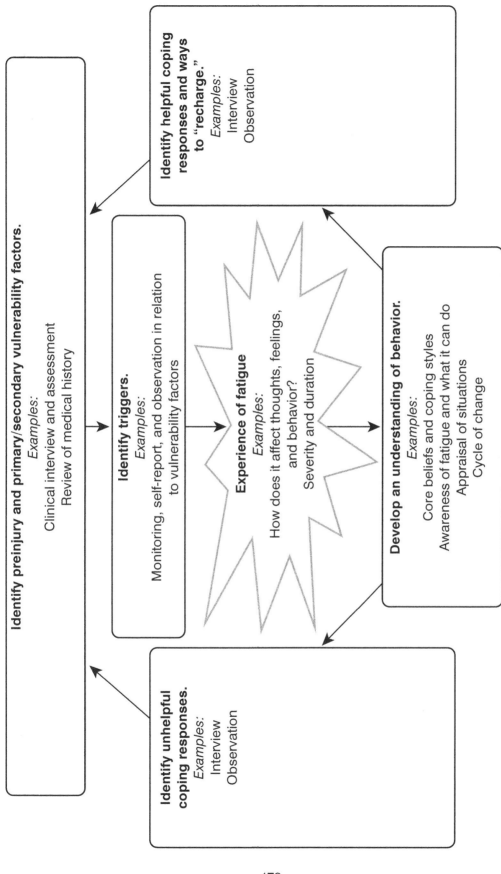

Identify helpful coping responses and ways to "recharge."
Examples:
Interview
Observation

Identify preinjury and primary/secondary vulnerability factors.
Examples:
Clinical interview and assessment
Review of medical history

Identify triggers.
Examples:
Monitoring, self-report, and observation in relation to vulnerability factors

Experience of fatigue
Examples:
How does it affect thoughts, feelings, and behavior?
Severity and duration

Develop an understanding of behavior.
Examples:
Core beliefs and coping styles
Awareness of fatigue and what it can do
Appraisal of situations
Cycle of change

Identify unhelpful coping responses.
Examples:
Interview
Observation

FIGURE 7.2. Using the model to guide assessment. Copyright © 2015 by The Oliver Zangwill Centre. Adapted by permission.

Raymont, & Grafman, 2010), as well as anxiety and depression (Wu, Barugh, Macleod, & Mead, 2014; Radman et al., 2012; Schnieders et al., 2012; Crosby et al., 2012). These are considered vulnerability factors in the fatigue model.

For people experiencing persistent fatigue following ABI, psychological and social consequences may be significant factors affecting their responses. Individuals are making adjustments to significant changes in their sense of themselves and their lives as a consequence of the ABI. One study proposed that poststroke fatigue (PSF) can be considered as due to a combination of organic brain lesion and psychosocial stress related to adjustment (Glader, Stegmayr, & Asplund, 2002). Self-efficacy, locus of control, coping styles, and social support appear to be associated with PSF and could be potential objectives for intervention (Wu et al., 2015). In addition, a lack of acknowledgment of PSF from others complicates coping and increases emotional distress (Eilertsen et al., 2013). A "coping hypothesis" has been proposed for fatigue following TBI, in response to increased effort in the face of reduced cognitive functioning (Cantor, Gordon, & Gumber, 2013; Ponsford et al., 2012). These studies suggest that fatigue management after ABI should incorporate psychosocial approaches, in addition to cognitive rehabilitation, pharmacological intervention, lifestyle changes, and environmental modifications.

FATIGUE MANAGEMENT STRATEGIES

There is no single, simple cure for fatigue following brain injury. For some people, fatigue improves over time; others may never feel that they can fully "recharge their batteries." However, it is possible to manage fatigue in order to make the best use of a client's available energy resources. As noted earlier, managing fatigue requires a variety of strategies in combination, to address the many interacting factors that may be contributing to it. Some strategies may seem like common sense, and clients may already be applying them. Taking the time to find out what works best for each person, and to help the person put some of these principles into consistent practice, should allow him or her to cope better with everyday activities. The clinical model can be used to guide intervention (see Figure 7.3).

Note that these strategies will not prevent people from feeling fatigued at all times, but they will help them to use their energy resources and abilities more effectively to support participation in their desired activities. For fatigue arising secondary to the cognitive, communication, and mood-related consequences of brain injury, many of the strategies described in other chapters of this workbook can be used to support management of fatigue.

Moreover, not every strategy works for every person, and knowing doesn't immediately lead to doing. This is why mediating factors were added to the clinical model (see Figure 7.1 and Handout 7.1). The use of behavioral experiments can help support people who may be ambivalent about certain management approaches in trying out techniques to see whether they work for them or not. For example, a person may believe that taking a break will mean achieving less, so the person may be reluctant to try pacing as a strategy. Discuss with this client what evidence would need to be collected to support this hypothesis. Then identify any alternative hypotheses (e.g., taking a break will mean fewer mistakes and won't affect how much gets done). Have the client try both approaches, and then ask him or her to reflect

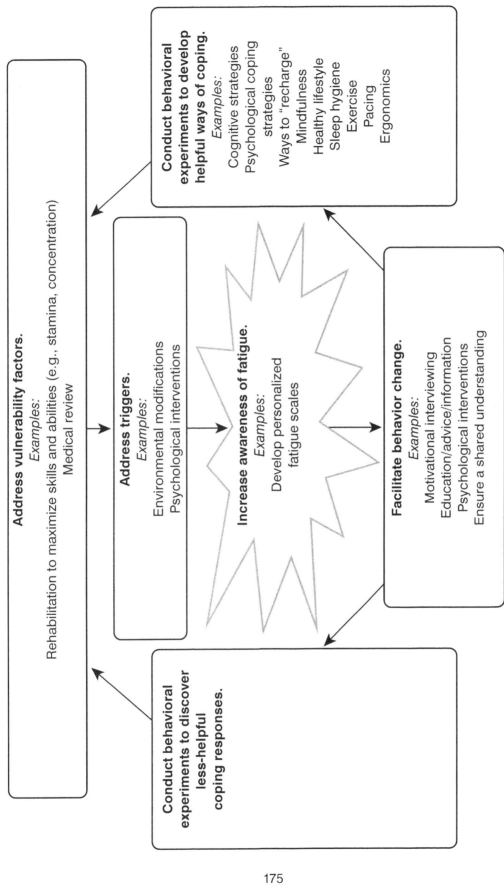

Address vulnerability factors.
Examples:
Rehabilitation to maximize skills and abilities (e.g., stamina, concentration)
Medical review

Conduct behavioral experiments to develop helpful ways of coping.
Examples:
Cognitive strategies
Psychological coping strategies
Ways to "recharge"
Mindfulness
Healthy lifestyle
Sleep hygiene
Exercise
Pacing
Ergonomics

Address triggers.
Examples:
Environmental modifications
Psychological interventions

Increase awareness of fatigue.
Examples:
Develop personalized fatigue scales

Facilitate behavior change.
Examples:
Motivational interviewing
Education/advice/information
Psychological interventions
Ensure a shared understanding

Conduct behavioral experiments to discover less-helpful coping responses.

FIGURE 7.3. Using the model to guide intervention. Copyright © 2015 by The Oliver Zangwill Centre. Adapted by permission.

on what happened and which hypothesis has gathered more evidence. This approach, taken from cognitive-behavioral therapy (CBT), is particularly useful not only for people who may feel ambivalent about trying out new ways of coping, but for those who may benefit from explicit evidence of what they have tried and what works best for them. More detail is given on behavioral experiments by Winegardner in Chapter 5, and by Ford in Chapter 8, of this book.

As noted throughout this chapter, fatigue management is not a linear process. Rather, we have found that it tends to fall into four main categories, which may overlap, repeat themselves, and interact with one another:

- Creating a shared understanding.
- Encouraging clients to monitor their level of energy/fatigue.
- Supporting clients in making the best use of their resources.
- Helping clients to develop ways to recharge their energy levels.

The descriptions below of activities and handouts have therefore been arranged under these headings.

Creating a Shared Understanding

What Is Fatigue?

One of the first things to do is to develop a shared understanding with clients of why they get fatigued and to help them acknowledge fatigue as a consequence of the injury, rather than as laziness! Other people need to understand this too. Making an analogy with something like a smartphone can be helpful. We need to ensure that our phones are charged enough to do the different tasks we may need to do in a day. These tasks may include making calls or texts, using the satellite navigation function, surfing the Internet, playing games, or taking photos. Certain tasks/functions can drain the battery on a smartphone really quickly, so we may need to plan to recharge our batteries during the day. We also need to keep an eye on the charge level throughout the day so we don't suddenly run out. A similar analogy may be a car's needing gasoline: We need to monitor the fuel gauge in relation to the travel we wish to undertake, to ensure we don't run out of gas.

Discuss the three different types of fatigue (physical, mental, and emotional) with clients, and ask which types they experience. Ask how each type feels for them and what impact it has. Listen to their language and try to use it when discussing their fatigue in later therapy sessions, to personalize intervention. Is there an analogy that works best for a particular client? It may be possible to create a personalized Likert fatigue/energy scale, using a client's descriptors to support his or her self-monitoring.

Explain to clients that fatigue is a personal experience that feels different for everyone. Begin by introducing Handout 7.1 as a way of making sense of how different aspects of fatigue can interact with one another. Explain that this may also indicate how their fatigue can be managed or reduced over time. Ask clients the following questions, and discuss their answers:

- What do you think makes you vulnerable to fatigue? (Answers may include deconditioning/loss of fitness, being slower to process information or more easily distracted, feeling stressed, or getting a poor night's sleep.)
- Which activities or situations may be potential triggers for you? (Answers may include busy environments, arguments, or tasks requiring lots of physical or cognitive effort.)
- What signs/symptoms may indicate that you are getting fatigued? (Answers may include aches and pains, feeling lightheaded, or visual problems.) What do other people notice?
- How do you respond when you are feeling fatigued? What impact does this have in the short term and over the longer term?
- What are the factors that might affect how you respond? (Answers may include low mood, lack of time, or the people to whom clients are responding.)

Now assist clients in starting to fill in sections of the formulation template in Handout 7.4, based on such preliminary discussions. What are the clients curious about? Where are the gaps in their knowledge? The process of completing Handout 7.4 may help develop a shared understanding and validation of their experience, and may be useful in explaining their fatigue to others.

Identifying Vulnerability Factors

With each client, work through Handout 7.5, which is a screening tool to identify factors that may be associated with the client's fatigue. There may be some you both know and some areas of uncertainty. Create an action plan together to explore areas of uncertainty. Consider whether the individual requires a medical review to consider primary fatigue factors, medication options, or management of associated conditions.

Identifying Triggers for Fatigue

The activities that trigger fatigue will be different for each individual. Commonly reported triggers include socializing, shopping, completing paperwork, and traveling. It may be helpful to use Handout 7.6 to discuss clients' different activities and the different kinds of energy (physical, mental, and emotional) they use in doing them. Activities can be added to the ones listed in this handout as required. Understanding that different activities and situations can lead to different types of fatigue helps when you and clients are thinking about planning and pacing what the clients need to do to recharge their energy levels.

Particular thoughts and particular situations may also be triggers for fatigue. It is helpful to discover what activities or situations are more fatiguing for clients, as well as which may be less fatiguing or actually energizing. Some people may easily identify triggers, while others may struggle. Use of a simple Likert scale (e.g., a scale where 10 = "full of energy" and 0 = "completely drained of energy"; try to use a client's own descriptions at the end-points) to rate energy levels before and after activities throughout the day may demonstrate this more clearly (see Handout 7.7). Monitoring over 1–2 weeks can be a starting point to help clients consider their triggers.

Some people find this intensity of monitoring difficult. In this case, monitoring levels of fatigue at consistent points in the day (e.g., 9:00 A.M., 1:00 P.M., 5:00 P.M., 9:00 P.M.), or before and after certain activities, can help clients to discover their personal triggers. Patterns (such as having more energy in the mornings) may emerge, but this is not always the case. Bear in mind that monitoring can be difficult for people with ABI, due to disrupted internal sensory processing, executive dysfunction, or simple forgetting. Some clients may need support to create their own fatigue scales before they can monitor their fatigue in more detail throughout the day.

Monitoring Energy/Fatigue Levels

In order to manage fatigue, clients need to be able to recognize when it is starting to build up. Handout 7.8 can be used to help clients consider how they know when they are getting fatigued; they can annotate the diagram with words or pictures. Often the signs and symptoms described are indicative of when their energy levels have been completely drained.

Some people may struggle to identify sensations, thoughts, feelings, and behaviors associated with their fatigue. This may be due either to poor self-monitoring or to loss of sensory awareness. In such cases, ask the clients what other people notice. In addition, what do you as a clinician observe, and what do family members or caregivers report observing? Supporting people in monitoring their own fatigue is a vital aspect of fatigue management, as clients need to be able to take action before they feel completely drained/exhausted.

It is usually helpful to then develop a simple but personalized "energy scale," as described in connection with identifying triggers. Sometimes it is possible to create a more detailed Likert scale, identifying how they feel at the different points on the scale. Sometimes it is more helpful just to create three main stages—"full of energy," "half-full," and "completely drained." In this case, a "traffic light" analogy can be useful, in which green represents full energy, yellow represents half-full, and red represents empty (see Handout 7.9). People have also used rulers, batteries, and jars as analogies of energy levels.

Although fatigue is a personal experience, others may notice signs of fatigue before the clients do, so ask these others what they notice too, to help clients create their scales. This will also help develop their awareness and understanding of the impact of fatigue.

The gingerbread person exercise will usually reveal how clients feel when they are completely exhausted. It is important to implement management strategies before this point, as many clients notice that their energy levels drain more rapidly when these levels drop below 50% charged/half-full. As a general rule, the 50% level is probably the most useful time for clients to take action and recharge their batteries, as often it is harder for them to take action when they are completely drained. Sometimes a client can work out the halfway point by using common sense, though discussion or observation and monitoring can help.

Making the Best Use of Available Resources

The Three P's: Pacing, Prioritizing, and Planning

Although pacing is commonly recommended for people experiencing fatigue, the recommendation is much easier to make than to implement. Few people, with or without brain injury, want to pace themselves; we all just want to get on with life! Pacing includes the following:

- Having regular breaks and/or using relaxation techniques.
- Planning our time and being organized.
- Prioritizing certain activities when we don't have enough energy for everything.
- Working within our available resources.
- Doing activities that may be energizing in between tasks that drain our energy.

Supporting clients in planning and prioritizing where they want and need to use their available energy can be tricky. Following monitoring, it may be possible to assign "energy points" to certain activities. An activity requiring more energy is given more points (e.g., reading a book may get 10 points, whereas chatting with a friend may get 3). Ask clients to imagine that they only have a certain number of points in a day, and to consider the following questions:

- How would you assign these points?
- What could you do to add to the available points (e.g., engaging in activities that recharge the batteries)?
- Do the same activities require the same points every time? Consider the impact of other factors, such as environment, context, or being around certain people.

Prioritizing involves asking clients to think about all the activities they have to do each day/week and to consider these questions:

- Which jobs are more important or essential?
- Which activities do you enjoy?
- Which tasks could you delegate to someone else?
- Could you do any activities less often or eliminate them altogether?

It is important for clients to strive for balance of activities between those that need to be done, and those that enable clients to feel a sense of pleasure or achievement in doing them. Ask the clients to identify all the activities they need to do and want to do, as well as to consider which activities could be done by someone else. Handout 7.10 can help clients consider this.

Planning time and being organized are vital to ensure that clients achieve the tasks they set out to do. Is there a consistent time of the day when they are at their best or when they feel fatigued? Encourage them to think about strategies that could support them in planning and organizing. What do others do? What might work best for them? Refer to strategies discussed in the chapters on attention, memory, and executive functions for ideas on how to plan and organize. You may need to review the use of external memory aids to support the clients in remembering what they need to do. They can use Handout 7.11 to plan activities into a weekly schedule.

Certain combinations of activities may work best (e.g., a physically demanding activity after a cognitively demanding task). What tasks can be inserted into each day to recharge a client's energy levels? In addition, encourage each client to allow some flexibility in the timetable, to allow for things that may just crop up or that have to be rescheduled at the last minute. Achieving a reasonable daily and weekly schedule may take time, but having a structured schedule reduces the effort of decision making "in the moment" and increases the likelihood of getting things done.

Sleep

Leading a healthy lifestyle is a foundation for any fatigue management approach. This incorporates getting a good night's sleep, eating a healthy diet, and getting appropriate exercise.

It makes sense that if clients have less sleep than they need, they will feel tired the following day. Getting enough good-quality sleep is an important aspect of managing fatigue. Common sleep complaints in people experiencing fatigue include the following:

- Difficulty initiating sleep.
- Difficulty maintaining sleep.
- Restless sleep with frequent dreams.
- Unrefreshing sleep.
- Excessive daytime sleepiness.

After brain injury, people may experience a range of sleep problems. Lying awake worrying or waking early in the morning may be indicative of a mood disorder, and so a psychological intervention may be required. A proportion of people will have a treatable sleep disorder, which may be either secondary to the injury or preexisting (e.g., sleep apnea). These disorders can be managed by a sleep center, so clients with sleep problems should discuss these with their GPs/PCPs to find out whether referral to a sleep center would be helpful. However, some sleep difficulties can be addressed through applying good sleep hygiene principles such as these:

- Creating a more consistent sleep–wake routine. The main goal is to try and help the brain know when to be alert and when to switch off. If this routine is severely disrupted, a client should focus first on establishing a more consistent waking pattern and getting out of bed at a certain time. If this time is very late in the morning, encourage the person to set an alarm (and get up at that time, regardless of how sleepy or fatigued the person feels) for 15 minutes earlier. When this time is successfully established, the person should set the alarm a further 15 minutes earlier, and so on, until an appropriate waking time is established. Clients should also avoid napping during the day, but if a nap is needed, then they should try to take it at a consistent point in the day (usually early afternoon).

- Ensuring that the bedroom is conducive to sleep by removing electronic devices, ensuring the right temperature, and providing a supportive mattress.
- Avoiding caffeine, nicotine, and alcohol within 6 hours of bedtime (Drake, Roehrs, Shambroom, & Roth, 2013).
- Avoiding vigorous exercise in the evening (although exercise at other times of day can promote good sleep; see below).
- Avoiding eating a heavy meal late in the evening.
- Establishing a relaxing bedtime routine.

Research evidence suggests that regular exposure to certain types of light may reduce levels of fatigue and daytime sleepiness (Sinclair, Ponsford, Taffe, Lockley, & Rajaratnam, 2014; Ponsford et al., 2012). It may also have a positive impact on mood and aspects of attention. Exposure to bright light on rising (e.g., natural daylight or a light box) will help set the body clock. Short-wavelength (blue) light therapy (at least 10,000 lux) has been demonstrated to be most effective for fatigue and daytime sleepiness. Sleep centers are good sources of support and advice regarding specific light sources and regimens for clients to use.

Exercise

Exercising improves the capacity to undertake physical activities. Some people report that physical exercise has a positive effect on their mental as well as their physical energy levels, and research shows that it can have a positive effect on mood. Exercise can also help with getting a better quality of sleep. Current U.K. and U.S. government guidelines recommend 30 minutes of moderately intense exercise (i.e., activity that makes the heart beat faster) five times a week to improve physical fitness. Before planning an exercise regimen for a client, however, consider whether medical, physical, and/or cognitive issues may have an impact on the client's participating in physical activity safely. Seek advice from the client's GP/PCP if either of you is uncertain. In the United Kingdom, there may be a GP referral scheme associated with local leisure centers that can be used as a starting point to enable participation in a supported exercise program.

Explore with clients ways in which they can incorporate physical activity into their everyday routines (e.g., using stairs rather than elevators, getting off the bus a stop earlier).

Nutrition

Eating the right kinds of food at regular times of day is essential to providing the body and brain with the energy it needs to do the things a person wants to do. As part of the assessment of fatigue, clients can be asked to keep a food diary for 1 week, to help identify dietary intake factors that may influence their energy levels. These may include skipping meals, drinking insufficient fluids, or relying on sugary foods or caffeine to "boost" energy levels. Also ask clients to consider other factors that may influence nutrition and hydration. These may include disruptions to senses (smell, taste, satiation, feeling a sense of hunger or thirst), mobility, ability to prepare meals, and/or memory and executive functions. Encouraging clients to ensure that their nutrition and hydration are sufficient to sustain energy levels will promote cognitive processes and mood in addition to physical functioning. A nutritionist or dietician may be able to offer more specific advice. In the United Kingdom, more information about healthy eating is available from a National Health Service webpage (*www.nhs.uk/Livewell/Goodfood/Pages/eight-tips-healthy-eating.aspx*). In the United States, the U.S. Department of Agriculture is the standard source of guidance (see, e.g., *www.nutrition.gov/smart-nutrition-101/myplate-resources*).

Strategies to Reduce Mental Effort

Many of the cognitive strategies identified in other chapters of this workbook can support people to manage their fatigue (e.g., using timetables and checklists to help keep on track; using external memory aids to reduce cognitive load; using the Goal Management Framework (GMF) and Time Pressure Management (TPM) to support planning and getting things done; allowing more time for tasks; and focusing on one task at a time). Use assessment results and other symptom questionnaires to identify difficulties and appropriate strategies to try out. Involve families/caregivers as much as possible.

Reducing errors through using such strategies can help boost self-confidence and thereby reduce fatigue secondary to low mood. Repeated practice is needed to consolidate and generalize strategy use.

Strategies to Manage Stress and Worry

Managing stress and worry is a significant drain on energy resources. Fatigue is one of the main criteria used in diagnosing depression. However, not everyone who experiences fatigue is depressed! Brain injury and its consequences can have a significant impact on mood and behavior; adjusting to and coping with the injury and its effects are really stressful experiences for everyone involved. Before vulnerability factors and triggers are identified, many people feel that fatigue is something they are unable to control, and this can lead them to feel helpless or hopeless. Clients' typical coping strategies can involve either trying to push themselves harder and so getting into a "boom–bust cycle" of doing too much and then collapsing with tiredness, or avoiding certain activities altogether. Feeling low, stressed, and worried can leave persons feeling extremely tired, even though they may feel they aren't doing anything. Equally, when people experience high levels of fatigue that stop them from doing what they want to do, they may report feeling low, frustrated, and irritable. These sequences can become vicious cycles, as noted earlier in this chapter, and family members may feel fatigued for these reasons as well. The evidence for psychosocial factors' being associated with fatigue and influencing behavioral responses is growing, and the role of psychosocial factors in adjusting to the consequences of ABI is well known. For some clients, this aspect of fatigue management can have a significant negative impact on their ability to put into practice information discussed with their therapists.

The following advice to clients can be used alongside the mood management strategies described by Ford in Chapter 8 to reduce stress and worry:

- Be realistic when planning: Pace activities to avoid the "boom–bust cycle," and break things down into smaller chunks.
- Attempt to reschedule activities for times when less fatigue is experienced; try not to dwell on things that haven't been achieved.
- Notice when things have gone well and acknowledge these achievements, perhaps by writing them down somewhere.
- Be aware of and acknowledge feelings and emotions, but try not to ruminate on or react to them. Mindfulness meditation may help (see Chapter 8).
- Plan time for pleasurable activities to boost self-esteem.
- Set realistic goals; acknowledge that it may not be possible to do as much as you could previously.

If clients are really struggling with mood, advise them to see their GPs/PCPs. Options may include medication, counseling, or psychotherapy such as CBT.

Clinicians may find it useful to use a mood screen to identify the presence of mood disorder that requires psychological or medical referral. For clients who struggle to implement lifestyle changes despite understanding and remembering the information, the mediating factors of the fatigue formulation may require particular attention. What meaning does fatigue hold for these clients? What coping styles are they using, and are these effective? What other factors may be influencing the clients' behavior? Consideration of where they are in the cycle of change and adjustment to their injury is necessary for many people with persistent fatigue, and use of motivational interviewing techniques may be appropriate at the contemplation stage in the cycle (Rollnick, Mason, & Butler, 1999).

Managing the Environment

To help each client make the best use of available mental and physical abilities, consider the physical, social, and cultural environment in which the person with fatigue is participating. Supporting individuals to consider the impact of the environment on their performance is one way to make sense of variability in performance. Being organized, planning ahead, and avoiding distractions can minimize the physical and mental effort that is required to complete an activity. The following suggestions to clients may help:

- Try to keep things in the same place, so that energy is not wasted in searching for things. Try to have "a place for everything and everything in its place."
- Organize workspaces; keep them as uncluttered as possible.

- Good lighting prevents eyestrain.
- Use labels/signs to help with finding things more easily.
- Think about turning off the TV or music when trying to concentrate on a task.
- Avoid interruptions from other people; if necessary, put a "Do Not Disturb" sign on the door.
- Consider making changes in some physical aspects of the environment (e.g., where things are stored), to save personal energy.

Having clear expectations (of both oneself and others) about performance and roles can also reduce worry and support planning.

Recharging Energy Levels

Helping clients find methods to recharge their energy levels quickly, so that they will have sufficient energy to do something later, is really important. This is particularly challenging when cognitive fatigue and emotional fatigue are significant. It is important to bear in mind that the choice of methods for doing this is a personal decision, because not everyone recharges in the same way. Also, how people recharge depends on what type of energy they have been using (physical, mental, or emotional). Handout 7.12 can help clients to consider what works best for them. Strategies may include the following:

- Taking a short "power nap" at the same time each day (but not after 4:00 P.M., as this can disrupt the sleep–wake cycle).
- Using relaxation techniques.
- Practicing mindfulness meditation or mindfulness-based stress reduction.
- Listening to music.
- Going for a walk, or otherwise getting some fresh air and exercise.
- Changing to a different type of activity (e.g., from a physical to a mental activity, or vice versa).
- Being around other people or being alone, depending on circumstances and personal preferences.
- Delegating/prioritizing activities.

People often need to experiment to find what works best for them. Encourage clients to add their own ideas of what works for them to their personal fatigue formulation.

BRINGING IT ALL TOGETHER

Support clients in using Handout 7.4 to complete their personalized fatigue formulation. Ask them to consider these questions:

- Pacing: What activities do you want to do, and what kind of energy does each activity need (physical, mental, emotional)?
- What can be done to reduce the energy needed for each activity?
- What can be done to recharge your batteries during the day?
- Which signs/symptoms may indicate that you are getting fatigued (i.e., reaching the 50% point on your personal fatigue scale)? Understanding these can enable you to take action before fatigue becomes completely overwhelming.
- Which factors might affect how you respond to fatigue? Knowing these factors can help you to make choices about how to manage the fatigue.
- What are the best ways to describe your fatigue to others—family, friends, colleagues, caregivers?

It may be best to have each client complete Handout 7.4 as you discover things in your work together. Both words (ideally, the individual's own words) and visual images can be used to create a personal formulation. Some people have gone on to create visual images or cue cards to help them monitor their fatigue and remember ways to manage it. Work with clients to identify how they are going to remember what they can do to manage their fatigue and share this understanding with others (families, friends, employers, colleagues, caregivers).

Clients may need frequent reassurance throughout this process. Finding out how to live with fatigue can be complicated, and it may take some time to work out the best way for each person. Although it may feel like an effort just to think about and implement these changes, over time they should become a more automatic part of clients' daily lives. They may still experience fatigue, but they should be able to participate in more activities more frequently and more successfully.

CASE STUDY

Karen was leading a hectic life as a flight attendant when, in her late 20s, she sustained a brain injury and spinal fractures in a road traffic accident. Despite attempts to return to the job she loved, overwhelming fatigue meant that she was unable to cope; she was diagnosed with chronic fatigue syndrome and fibromyalgia, and had to return to living with her parents after the breakdown of her marriage. The problems Karen faced in dealing with her fatigue, and some of her goals and strategies for dealing with these problems, are described in Table 7.1.

TABLE 7.1. Dealing with Karen's Fatigue-Related Challenges

Challenges	Goals and strategies	Context for rehabilitation
Low mood, rumination, self-criticism; anxiety, irritability, anger; loss of confidence; avoidant coping style Karen described negative repeating cycles of striving hard to do things, experiencing failure, asking herself why she bothered, feeling extremely low in mood, and then having to pick herself up again. *Divided attention and executive dysfunction* Karen had been trying to slow herself down a bit, but was struggling with the pace of life. She felt overwhelmed and perceived everything as effortful.	Overall goal: To feel more in control of fatigue. To understand factors influencing fatigue: • Thorough assessment identified cognitive impairments, physical factors (comorbid health condition), emotional factors, sleep disturbance, and past experiences. • Karen was referred to an endocrinologist. To feel less frustrated about fatigue: • Personalized formulation increased Karen's understanding and allowed her experience of fatigue to be shared. • Better understanding reduced Karen's anxiety. • Identifying strategies collaboratively further reduced her frustration. To manage fatigue and make best use of resources: • Memory and planning strategies • GMF (to support decision making) • A mindfulness- and compassion-focused approach (to manage psychological distress) • CBT (to challenge negative automatic thoughts) • Skills building • Managing the environment Karen reported a greater sense of control, rather than feeling as if fatigue had taken over her life. She developed a personalized "fatigue battery" to enable her to monitor her energy levels more effectively "in the moment."	Karen wanted to learn how to do things differently to enable independent living, socializing, and vocational development. Karen had a period of inpatient rehabilitation, which addressed the practical consequences of physical fatigue for basic activities of daily living. Energy conservation approaches, nutrition, sleep hygiene, structuring, and pacing activities enabled independence. Learning undertaken during intensive neuropsychological rehabilitation allowed Karen to start reengaging with meaningful activities, which fatigue had prevented her from enjoying for some time. For instance, Karen loved having her niece and nephew to visit, but found it hard to cope with two energetic youngsters. Information from Karen's fatigue formulation was used to determine her levels of activity tolerance. She was helped to plan a visit, using this information and her cognitive strategies. • A structured timetable for the visit was devised, allowing time for fun activities with the children, and building in rest periods. Karen used her artistic skills to present this timetable in the form of a party invitation. • A carefully paced schedule was planned for the week before the visit, to allow time for preparation and rest. Mindfulness meditation was built into each day, and the plan allowed time for Karen to bake a cake for the visit—an activity she had valued highly before her injury. • A behavioral experiment approach was used before and after the visit. "Emergency" strategies were planned in advance in case Karen became overwhelmed. Following a successful visit, Karen used a similar approach to plan a weekend away visiting a friend. After her "graduation" from the rehabilitation program, Karen returned to the service for further input. She was supported to make sense of her injury through the lens of fatigue, and identify new "rules" for living her life consistent with her values. She was ultimately able to plan a trip abroad to do volunteer work, before engaging in a course of vocational study.

REFERENCES

Cantor, J. B., Ashman, T., Bushnik, T., Cai, X., Farrell-Carnahan, L., Gumber, S., . . . Dijkers, M. (2014). Systematic review of interventions for fatigue after traumatic brain injury: A NIDRR Traumatic Brain Injury Model Systems Study. *Journal of Head Trauma Rehabilitation, 29*(6), 490–497.

Cantor, J. B., Gordon, W., & Gumber, S. (2013). What is post-TBI fatigue? *NeuroRehabilitation, 32*(4), 875–883.

Crosby, G. A., Munshi, S., Karat, A. S., Worthington, E., & Lincoln, N. (2012). Fatigue after stroke: frequency and effect on daily life. *Disability and Rehabilitation, 34*(8), 633–637.

Drake, C., Roehrs, T., Shambroom, J., & Roth, T. (2013). Caffeine effects on sleep taken 0, 3, or 6 hours before going to bed. *Journal of Clinical Sleep Medicine, 9*(11), 1195–1200.

Duncan, F., Wu, S., & Mead, G. E. (2012). Frequency and natural history of fatigue after stroke: A systematic review of longitudinal studies. *Journal of Psychosomatic Research, 73*(1), 18–27.

Eilertsen, G., Ormstad, H., & Kirkevold, M. (2013). Experiences of post-stroke fatigue: Qualitative meta-synthesis. *Journal of Advanced Nursing, 69*(3), 514–525.

Elbers, R. G., Rietberg, M. B., Wegen, E. E. H., Verhoef, J., Kramer, S. F., Terwee, C. B., & Kwakkel, G. (2012). Self-report fatigue questionnaires in multiple sclerosis, Parkinson's disease and stroke: A systematic review of measurement properties. *Quality of Life Research, 21*(6), 925–944.

Elovic, E. P., Dobrovic, N. M., & Fellus, J. L. (2005). Fatigue after traumatic brain injury. In J. DeLuca (Ed.), *Fatigue as a window to the brain* (pp. 91–105). Cambridge, MA: MIT Press.

Glader, E. L., Stegmayr, B., & Asplund, K. (2002). Post-stroke fatigue: A 2-year follow-up study of stroke patients in Sweden. *Stroke, 33*(5), 1327–1333.

Hoang, C. L. N., Sall, J. Y., Mandigout, S., Hamonet, J., Macian-Montor, F., & Daviet, J.-C. (2012). Physical factors associated with fatigue after stroke: An exploratory study. *Topics in Stroke Rehabilitation, 19*(5), 369–376.

Kluger, B. M., Krupp, L. B., & Enoka, R. M. (2013). Fatigue and fatigability in neurologic illnesses: Proposal for a unified taxonomy. *Neurology, 80*(4), 409–416.

Krupp, L. B., La Rocca, N. G., Muir-Nash, J., & Steinberg, A. D. (1989). The Fatigue Severity Scale: Application to patients with multiple sclerosis and systemic lupus erythematosus. *Archives of Neurology, 46*, 1121–1123.

Kutlubaev, M. A., Mead, G. E., & Lerdal, A. (2015). Fatigue after stroke: Perspectives and future directions. *International Journal of Stroke, 10*(3), 280–281.

Lerdal, A., Bakken, L. N., Kouwenhoven, S. E., Pedersen, G., Kirkevold, M., Finset, A., & Kim, H. S. (2009). Post-stroke fatigue: A review. *Journal of Pain and Symptom Management, 38*(6), 928–949.

Malley, D., Wheatcroft, J., & Gracey, F. (2014). Fatigue after ABI: A model to guide clinical management. *Advances in Clinical Neuroscience and Rehabilitation, 14*(2), 17–19.

Miller, K. K., Combs, S. A., Van Puymbroeck, M., Altenburger, P. A., Kean, J., Dierks, T. A., & Schmid, A. A. (2013). Fatigue and pain: Relationships with physical performance and patient beliefs after stroke. *Topics in Stroke Rehabilitation, 20*(4), 347–355.

Mills, R. J., Pallant, J. F., Koufali, M., Sharma, A., Day, S., Tennant, A., & Young, C. A. (2012). Validation of the Neurological Fatigue Index for Stroke (NFI-Stroke). *Health and Quality of Life Outcomes, 10*, 51.

Pardini, M., Krueger, F., Raymont, V., & Grafman, J. (2010). Ventromedial prefrontal cortex modulates fatigue after penetrating traumatic brain injury. *Neurology, 74*(9), 749–754.

Ponsford, J. L., & Sinclair, K. L. (2014). Sleep and fatigue following traumatic brain injury. *Psychiatric Clinics of North America, 37*(1), 77–89.

Ponsford, J. L., Ziino, C., Parcell, D. L., Shekleton, J. A., Roper, M., Redman, J. R., . . . Rajaratnam,

S. M. W. (2012). Fatigue and sleep disturbance following traumatic brain injury: Their nature, causes, and potential treatments. *Journal of Head Trauma Rehabilitation, 27*(3), 224–233.

Radman, N., Staub, F., Aboulafia-Brakha, T., Berney, A., Bogousslavsky, J., & Annoni, J.-M. (2012). Post-stroke fatigue following minor infarcts: A prospective study. *Neurology, 79*(14), 1422–1427.

Rollnick, S., Mason, P., & Butler, C. C. (1999). *Health behaviour change: A guide for practitioners.* London: Churchill Livingstone.

Ronnback, L., & Johansson, B. (2012). *Long-lasting mental fatigue after traumatic brain injury or stroke: A new perspective.* Saarbrucken, Germany: Lambert Academic.

Schnieders, J., Willemsen, D., & De Boer, H. (2012). Factors contributing to chronic fatigue after traumatic brain injury. *Journal of Head Trauma Rehabilitation, 27*(6), 404–412.

Sinclair, K. L., Ponsford, J. L., Taffe, J., Lockley, S. W., & Rajaratnam, S. M. (2014). Randomized controlled trial of light therapy for fatigue following traumatic brain injury. *Neurorehabilitation and Neural Repair, 28*(4), 303–313.

Wu, S., Barugh, A. J., Macleod, M., & Mead, G. E. (2014). Psychological associations of poststroke fatigue: A systematic review and meta-analysis. *Stroke, 45*(6), 1778–1783.

Wu, S., Mead, G., Macleod, M., & Chalder, T. (2015). Model of understanding fatigue after stroke. *Stroke, 46*(3), 893–898.

Model of Fatigue after Brain Injury

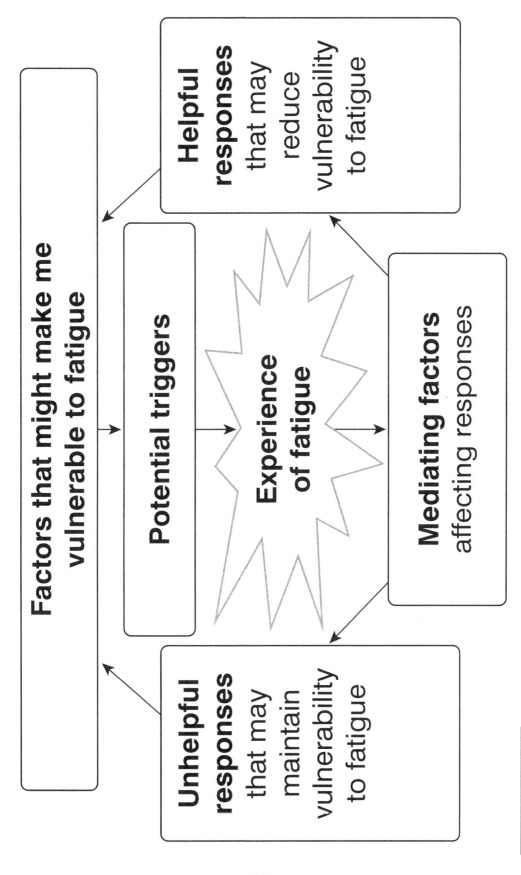

From *The Brain Injury Rehabilitation Workbook*, edited by Rachel Winson, Barbara A. Wilson, and Andrew Bateman. Copyright © 2017 The Guilford Press. Permission to photocopy this handout is granted to purchasers of this book for personal use or for use with individual clients (see copyright page for details). Purchasers can download additional copies of this handout (see the box at the end of the table of contents).

What Is Fatigue?

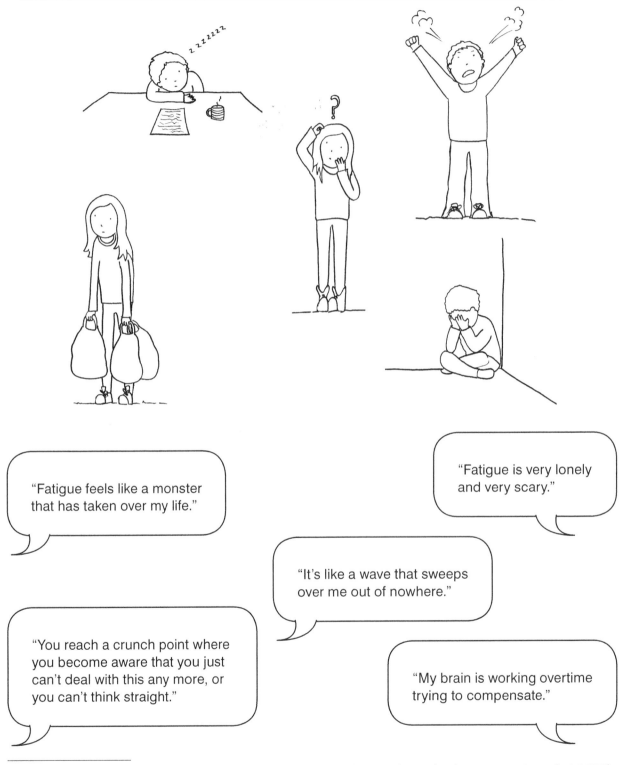

"Fatigue feels like a monster that has taken over my life."

"Fatigue is very lonely and very scary."

"It's like a wave that sweeps over me out of nowhere."

"You reach a crunch point where you become aware that you just can't deal with this any more, or you can't think straight."

"My brain is working overtime trying to compensate."

From *The Brain Injury Rehabilitation Workbook*, edited by Rachel Winson, Barbara A. Wilson, and Andrew Bateman. Copyright © 2017 The Guilford Press. Permission to photocopy this handout is granted to purchasers of this book for personal use or for use with individual clients (see copyright page for details). Purchasers can download additional copies of this handout (see the box at the end of the table of contents).

Fatigue Management Questionnaire

Please answer the following questions by circling a number on each 1–10 scale (1 = none at all, 10 = a lot).

Questions	Responses									
A. Do you know what contributes to your fatigue?	1	2	3	4	5	6	7	8	9	10
B. How much does fatigue worry/concern/distress/annoy/frustrate you?	1	2	3	4	5	6	7	8	9	10
C. How well are you able to manage your fatigue?	1	2	3	4	5	6	7	8	9	10
D. How much control do you feel you have over your fatigue?	1	2	3	4	5	6	7	8	9	10
E. How much is fatigue interfering with your ability to participate in everyday activities (over the past 2 weeks)?	1	2	3	4	5	6	7	8	9	10
How do you currently manage your fatigue?										
Do you have any specific questions or concerns you wish to discuss?										

From *The Brain Injury Rehabilitation Workbook*, edited by Rachel Winson, Barbara A. Wilson, and Andrew Bateman. Copyright © 2017 The Guilford Press. Permission to photocopy this handout is granted to purchasers of this book for personal use or for use with individual clients (see copyright page for details). Purchasers can download additional copies of this handout (see the box at the end of the table of contents).

Fatigue Formulation

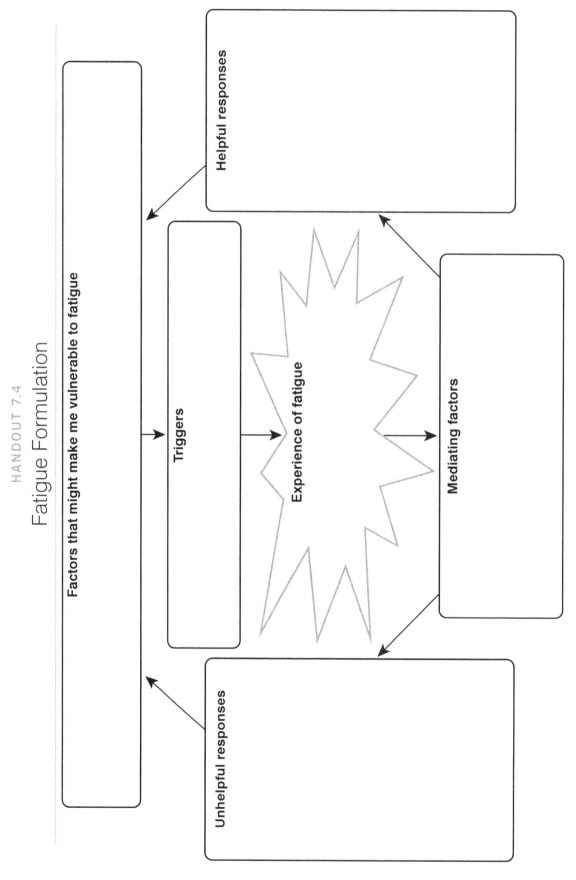

Factors that might make me vulnerable to fatigue

Helpful responses

Triggers

Experience of fatigue

Mediating factors

Unhelpful responses

From *The Brain Injury Rehabilitation Workbook*, edited by Rachel Winson, Barbara A. Wilson, and Andrew Bateman. Copyright © 2017 The Guilford Press. Permission to photocopy this handout is granted to purchasers of this book for personal use or for use with individual clients (see copyright page for details). Purchasers can download additional copies of this handout (see the box at the end of the table of contents).

Screening Tool

Fatigue

- ☐ Previous intervention and information?
- ☐ Onset and duration?
- ☐ Any patterns? Worse in A.M. or P.M., or neither?
- ☐ Reported triggers?
- ☐ Reported "refreshing" activities?
- ☐ Current tolerances for activity?
- ☐ Awareness of signs of fatigue/ability to monitor tiredness?
- ☐ Do others understand the client's fatigue?

Fatigue Indicators

- ☐ Fatigue scale
- ☐ Other measures (list): _____

_____

Sleep

- ☐ Regular sleep and wake times?
- ☐ Average hours of sleep?
- ☐ Waking early/difficulty getting to sleep?
- ☐ Feel refreshed on waking?
- ☐ Need naps during the day?
- ☐ Other factors affecting sleep quality and duration (e.g., snoring, urinary frequency during night)?

Endocrine Functioning

- ☐ Brain areas implicated: _____
- ☐ Sleep–wake cycle disruption?
- ☐ Altered temperature regulation?
- ☐ Altered appetite?

(continued)

From *The Brain Injury Rehabilitation Workbook*, edited by Rachel Winson, Barbara A. Wilson, and Andrew Bateman. Copyright © 2017 The Guilford Press. Permission to photocopy this handout is granted to purchasers of this book for personal use or for use with individual clients (see copyright page for details). Purchasers can download additional copies of this handout (see the box at the end of the table of contents).

☐ Ability to sense hunger/thirst?

☐ Evidence of significant weight loss or gain?

☐ Changes to skin condition/sexual functioning/menstruation?

☐ Previous investigations?

Physical and Medical Factors

☐ Side effects of medication?

☐ Medication to improve sleep or increase arousal?

☐ Presence of pain?

☐ Comorbid conditions (e.g., anemia, diabetes, chronic fatigue syndrome)?

☐ Presence of motor dysfunction?

☐ Current physical fitness?

Mood-Related Factors

☐ Presence of mood disorder (e.g., anxiety, depression, PTSD)?

☐ Psychological drives?

☐ Mood scale score (indicate which scale used):

Cognitive Factors

☐ Presence of reduced speed of processing or attentional difficulties?

☐ Presence of memory deficits?

☐ Presence of executive dysfunction?

Sensory Factors

☐ Presence of visual disturbance?

☐ Presence of auditory disturbance?

☐ Changes to sense of taste/smell?

☐ Changes to tactile sensation?

☐ Changes to vestibular function and proprioception?

☐ Sensory profile/preferences?

(continued)

Environmental Factors

☐ Physical (motor and sensory) and cognitive demands?

☐ Social/cultural factors?

☐ Lifestyle factors (e.g., diet, fitness)?

Fatigue Management Questionnaire Ratings

See Handout 7.3 (1 = none; 10 = a lot).

A. Knowledge of factors contributing to fatigue? ____

B. Level of worry/concern/distress/frustration associated with fatigue? ____

C. Ability to manage their fatigue? ____

D. Sense of control over fatigue? ____

E. Impact on activity level? ____

Client's Goals

_____

_____

_____

_____

_____

_____

_____

_____

_____

Additional Recommendations

☐ Need for endocrine investigations?

☐ Need for sleep clinic referral?

☐ Need for review by consultant in neurorehabilitation?

☐ Need for review by neuropsychiatrist?

Fatigue Triggers

Place a tick in each column against the type of energy you use for each activity.

Activity	Physical energy	Mental energy	Emotional energy
Personal care			
• Getting up			
• Getting washed			
• Getting dressed			
• Grooming			
• Toileting			
• Medication			
• Eating/drinking			
• Indoor mobility			
• Outdoor mobility			
• Getting on/off:			
o Bed			
o Chair			
o Toilet			
o Bath			
Domestic tasks			
• Hot drinks			
• Meal preparation:			
o Breakfast			
o Lunch/snack			
o Main meal			

(continued)

From *The Brain Injury Rehabilitation Workbook*, edited by Rachel Winson, Barbara A. Wilson, and Andrew Bateman. Copyright © 2017 The Guilford Press. Permission to photocopy this handout is granted to purchasers of this book for personal use or for use with individual clients (see copyright page for details). Purchasers can download additional copies of this handout (see the box at the end of the table of contents).

Activity	Physical energy	Mental energy	Emotional energy
• Laundry			
• Ironing			
• Money management			
• Cleaning			
Community tasks			
• Shopping			
• Driving			
• Use of public transport:			
o Taxis			
o Buses			
o Trains			
• Finding way around			
• Crossing roads			
Miscellaneous			
• Dealing with correspondence			
• Completing forms			
• Dealing with emergencies			
• Child care			
• Planning outings or holidays			
• Socializing (meals, parties)			
• Having conversations with people			

Fatigue Diary

Start and finish times	Activities completed	Fatigue level before	Fatigue level after	Difference between after and before (in points)	Factors influencing fatigue during activities
		(0 = no fatigue, 10 = worst fatigue possible)			(e.g., mood, hunger, sleep)

From *The Brain Injury Rehabilitation Workbook*, edited by Rachel Winson, Barbara A. Wilson, and Andrew Bateman. Copyright © 2017 The Guilford Press. Permission to photocopy this handout is granted to purchasers of this book for personal use or for use with individual clients (see copyright page for details). Purchasers can download additional copies of this handout (see the box at the end of the table of contents).

How Does It Feel?

Write or draw on the diagram how fatigue makes you feel.

What happens to your thinking, senses, movement, mood, and ability to communicate?

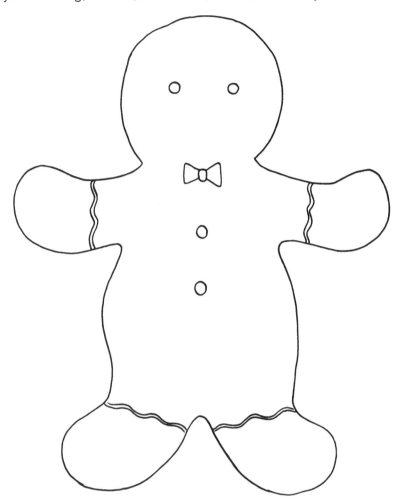

What does your fatigue look like to others?

From *The Brain Injury Rehabilitation Workbook*, edited by Rachel Winson, Barbara A. Wilson, and Andrew Bateman. Copyright © 2017 The Guilford Press. Permission to photocopy this handout is granted to purchasers of this book for personal use or for use with individual clients (see copyright page for details). Purchasers can download additional copies of this handout (see the box at the end of the table of contents).

My Fatigue Traffic Light

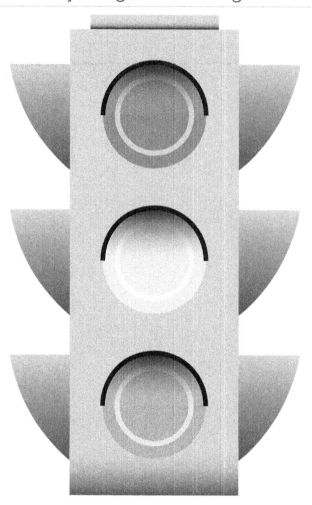

Indicate on the picture:

Red light: How does it feel when you have no energy at all? What do you do then?

Yellow light: How does it feel when you are a little bit tired? What do you do then?

Green light: How does it feel when you are full of energy? What do you do then?

From *The Brain Injury Rehabilitation Workbook*, edited by Rachel Winson, Barbara A. Wilson, and Andrew Bateman. Copyright © 2017 The Guilford Press. Permission to photocopy this handout is granted to purchasers of this book for personal use or for use with individual clients (see copyright page for details). Purchasers can download additional copies of this handout (see the box at the end of the table of contents).

The Art of Delegation

Consider all the things you currently spend time and energy doing. Now consider which column you could list them in below. Use this handout to help you plan and prioritize where you want and need to use your energy.

Things I have to do	Things I would like to do	Things someone else could do	Things that could be done if I have energy left over!

From *The Brain Injury Rehabilitation Workbook*, edited by Rachel Winson, Barbara A. Wilson, and Andrew Bateman. Copyright © 2017 The Guilford Press. Permission to photocopy this handout is granted to purchasers of this book for personal use or for use with individual clients (see copyright page for details). Purchasers can download additional copies of this handout (see the box at the end of the table of contents).

Weekly Timetable

	Monday	Tuesday	Wednesday	Thursday	Friday	Saturday	Sunday
Morning							
Afternoon							
Evening							

From *The Brain Injury Rehabilitation Workbook*, edited by Rachel Winson, Barbara A. Wilson, and Andrew Bateman. Copyright © 2017 The Guilford Press. Permission to photocopy this handout is granted to purchasers of this book for personal use or for use with individual clients (see copyright page for details). Purchasers can download additional copies of this handout (see the box at the end of the table of contents).

Recharging Different Types of Energy

Physical energy	Mental/cognitive energy	Emotional energy
Refill my energy levels/reduce effort by:	Refill my energy levels/reduce effort by:	Refill my energy levels by:

From *The Brain Injury Rehabilitation Workbook*, edited by Rachel Winson, Barbara A. Wilson, and Andrew Bateman. Copyright © 2017 The Guilford Press. Permission to photocopy this handout is granted to purchasers of this book for personal use or for use with individual clients (see copyright page for details). Purchasers can download additional copies of this handout (see the box at the end of the table of contents).

CHAPTER 8

Mood

Catherine Longworth Ford

We all have a range of basic emotions, such as fear, anger, sadness, surprise, disgust, and happiness. Experiencing these emotions, associating them with particular triggers, and controlling our responses to them involve a number of different areas of the brain working together. A brain injury can damage one or more of these areas or the connections between them, leading to a range of emotional changes, such as feeling more irritable, apathetic, restless, or excited than normal. Survivors of brain injury may also have difficulties inhibiting their emotional responses; they may find themselves crying or laughing with less control than before. Changes in emotion can become much more rapid, so that it becomes harder to think and solve problems. Brain injury causes some survivors to have difficulties understanding the emotions of others, which is likely to affect their relationships. On top of this, the survivors' normal strategies for coping with difficult situations and emotions (such as talking to friends or problem solving) may not work as well as before, due to other problems caused by brain injury. This can mean that they face different and difficult emotions, without feeling that they have effective ways to cope with them. They may also find it hard to cope with the difficult life situations that result from brain injury, such as becoming aware of impairments caused by the injury, not being able to work, or having problems in their relationships.

Many people with brain injury thus start to feel less good about themselves. Understandably they may become depressed, anxious, or angry about their situation, or feel guilty about the impact of their injury on those close to them. Taken together, the emotional changes, changes in control, and changes in coping responses (or lack of such responses) to the situation can start to affect everyday life and rehabilitation, leading to difficulties such as social withdrawal or aggression. It is important for survivors and those around them to know that it is possible to tackle problems with emotions and coping after brain injury.

Developing an understanding of these problems, recognizing the early signs of rising emotions, and using strategies to prevent difficulties can help clients with brain injury feel more in control and improve their emotional well-being.

THEORETICAL BACKGROUND, MODELS, AND EVIDENCE

A large proportion of people with acquired brain injury (ABI) develop clinically significant mood disorders. At least a third of those who survive stroke develop depression or anxiety (Hackett & Pickles, 2014). A third of those with traumatic brain injury (TBI) are reported to have emotional difficulties between 6 months and a year after injury (Bowen, Chamberlain, Tennant, Neumann, & Conner, 1999), and 44% develop two or more mood disorders, with the most common being depression and anxiety (Hibbard, Uysal, Kepler, Bogdany, & Silver, 1998). Mood disorder is associated with greater functional impairments after stroke (Parikh et al., 1990; Pohjasvaara, Vataja, Leppävuori, Kaste, & Erkinjuntti, 2001; Sinyor et al., 1986), as well as with increased caregiver strain (Anderson, Linto, & Stewart-Wynne, 1995). Post-stroke depression has also been associated with increased mortality (House, Knapp, Bamford, & Vail, 2001).

In the United Kingdom, a "Stepped Care approach" has been recommended in stroke services to address the scale of psychological difficulties after stroke, including mood disorders such as depression and anxiety (NHS Improvement—Stroke, 2011). To date, the Stepped Care approach has not been applied to rehabilitation for people with other types of ABI, such as TBI, although the interventions involved can also be used to support people with these injuries.

The Stepped Care approach provides psychological support according to clients' level of need, starting with simple interventions and progressing to more complex interventions as required. Simple interventions that can be provided by peers or rehabilitation staff are offered first to everyone (Level 1 psychological support). These interventions, such as help with problem solving and goal setting, may be sufficient to support people who are not clinically anxious or depressed in coping with their stroke and its consequences. More complex interventions, such as support with mindfulness exercises, are then offered to people who are found to have mild to moderate difficulties with depression or anxiety (Level 2 psychological support). These may be provided by nonpsychologist stroke specialist staff members, supervised by a specialist clinical psychologist or clinical neuropsychologist. The most complex interventions are provided by specialist clinical psychologists, clinical neuropsychologists, or neuropsychiatrists to people with severe and persistent mood disorders following stroke; such interventions include cognitive-behavioral therapy (CBT) and therapeutic approaches (Level 3 psychological support). The adoption of a Stepped Care approach to mood difficulties after stroke provides opportunities for rehabilitation staff to develop an understanding of the consequences of stroke for mood, together with skills in offering interventions to reduce symptoms of depression or anxiety.

To make sense of problems with mood after brain injury, it can help to understand why people respond differently even to the same situations; how emotions such as sadness, anxiety, or anger can become problematic; and what might help when this is the case. How the changes caused by brain injury affect a person's sense of identity is another key factor to understand in making sense of changes in mood after brain injury (see Gracey, Prince, & Winson, Chapter 9, this volume).

People have very different emotional responses to the same situations, suggesting that their memories and interpretations of situations play an important role in determining how they feel. The cognitive model (Beck, Rush, Shaw, & Emery, 1979; Greenberger & Padesky, 2015) suggests that our interpretations of what is going on around us can drive our emotional, physical, and behavioral responses to situations. For example, if we hear a noise in the night and interpret it as being caused by a pet, we are likely to remain calm and sleepy and stay in bed. If we think it is a burglar, however, we may feel scared or angry and go into a fight-or-flight response, ready to call the police. The cognitive model explains that people can respond to the same situation differently as a result of the way they think about it, which is influenced by the beliefs and assumptions they have developed throughout life from the experiences they have had. For example, people who tend to believe that others treat them badly may be more likely than people who tend to believe that others treat them well, to interpret the noise as being caused by a burglar.

CBT, based on the cognitive model, is a talking therapy that uses a range of techniques to help people overcome common problems, such as depression or anxiety disorders. It helps people identify and test the kinds of thoughts that maintain these disorders (e.g., "Nothing will ever go right for me" or "What if I can't cope?") and develop and test more helpful thoughts (e.g., "Although lots of things have been difficult, I am progressing well in rehabilitation"). Figure 8.1 offers an illustration of the CBT cycle of thoughts, feelings, physical sensations, and actions, and Handout 8.1 is a version of this illustration that can be shared with clients and families.* Handout 8.2 explains the components of the cycle in more detail.

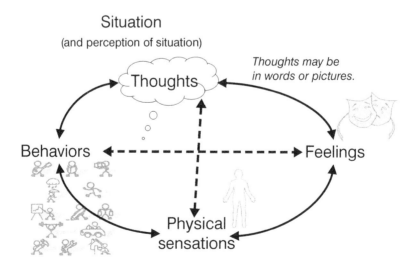

FIGURE 8.1. The cognitive-behavioral therapy (CBT) cycle.

---

* All handouts are at the end of the chapter.

There is promising evidence that CBT can be useful in reducing symptoms of depression or anxiety in people with ABI (Waldron, Casserly, & O'Sullivan, 2013). A number of case studies (Gracey, Oldham, & Kritzinger, 2007; Dewar & Gracey, 2007) and randomized controlled trials (Ashman, Cantor, Tsaousides, Spielman, & Gordon, 2014; Fann et al., 2015) support the efficacy of CBT as a treatment for depression after TBI. More research on CBT for people with ABI is required, however, particularly on CBT for survivors of stroke. The first randomized controlled trial of CBT for poststroke depression failed to find a significant benefit of CBT (Lincoln & Flannaghan, 2003). This may have been due to small sample size, or it may mean that CBT must be augmented and individually tailored to ensure effectiveness in the context of stroke (Broomfield et al., 2011).

Theories of stress and coping (e.g., Lazarus & Folkman, 1987) suggest that one reason people differ in their emotional responses relates to their individual interpretations of how a situation affects their ability to achieve goals they care about, given the resources they have available. A situation that we think poses a manageable challenge to our goals may increase our motivational drive; a situation we see as threatening our goals may make us feel stressed; a situation we see as leading to the loss of our goals may make us feel depressed. The coping strategies we employ in a situation reflect this appraisal. For example, we may respond to a challenge by redoubling our efforts, to a threat by seeking support to help us tackle a situation, or to a loss by comforting ourselves. After brain injury, some appraisals of the situation and coping strategies appear to be more helpful than others. For example, seeing oneself as having control over the situation rather than being controlled by it is associated with better emotional well-being after TBI (Moore & Stambrook, 1992), and less use of avoidance or wishful thinking predicts better psychosocial functioning (Malia, Powell, & Torode, 1995).

Compassion-focused therapy (CFT; Gilbert, 2000, 2010a, 2010b) suggests that to achieve emotional well-being there must be a balance among three evolutionary emotional systems, which are described and illustrated in Handout 8.3:

1. A "threat system," which equips us to survive situations that could endanger us by evoking powerful negative emotions that are hard to ignore, such as fear, anger, or disgust.
2. A "drive system," which pushes us to acquire what we need by evoking our feelings of motivation and desire.
3. A "soothing, compassionate system," which enables us to reduce our sense of threat and benefit from supportive relationships with others by evoking our feelings of contentment, kindness, and calm.

Without this balance, one set of emotions may dominate the others. For example, when life has involved abuse or trauma, the balance can become tipped toward negative emotional responses to threat, resulting in shame, self-criticism, and little or no sense of well-being. Even if someone had strong emotional well-being before brain injury, the difficulties of regulating the fast route to emotion after frontal lobe damage (described later) may tip the balance toward more negative, threat-based emotions and fewer positive emotions linked to self-acceptance, contentment, or motivational drive. The aim of CFT is to help people struggling with shame and self-criticism to develop self-compassion and compassion toward others, in order to reduce their sense of threat. There is promising evidence that CFT increases self-reassurance and reduces the self-criticism, depression, and anxiety that survivors can suffer after brain injury (Ashworth, Clarke, Jones, Jennings, & Longworth, 2015).

In addition to understanding how emotions can become problematic and what might help, it can be useful to understand positive emotions and ways to increase happiness and well-being. Proponents of positive psychology (e.g., Seligman, 2002) seek to understand why happy people are happy and how to increase happiness. They suggest that we can experience three different types of happiness through experiencing pleasure ("the pleasant life"), making full use of personal strengths in everyday life ("the engaged life"), and using these strengths in pursuit of a higher purpose ("the meaningful life"). Seligman and colleagues have developed and tested a number of interventions designed to increase happiness and well-being. The "three good things" intervention involves recording three things that went well each day and considering why they went well over the course of a week. The "using signature strengths in a different way" intervention involves identifying and using one key character strength each day for a week (Seligman, Steen, Park, & Peterson, 2005). In an online randomized controlled trial, Seligman's group found that these two interventions increased happiness and decreased depression compared to baseline after 1 month, and that these benefits lasted for at least 6 months (Seligman et al., 2005). Evans (2011) has proposed that the positive psychology approach is relevant to, and consistent with, brain injury rehabilitation. He suggests that people with ABI may benefit from the use of positive psychology interventions (modified to include support for cognitive impairments if necessary), and that it would be helpful to explore whether assessment of character strengths is useful after ABI. Research is required, however, to test whether the use of positive psychology interventions reduces depression and increases happiness after ABI.

NEUROANATOMY OF MOOD

Key parts of the brain involved in emotional responses and regulation are illustrated in Figure 8.2, and Handout 8.4 is a version of this figure with simplified labels that can be given to clients. The limbic system is a primitive set of interconnected areas involved with

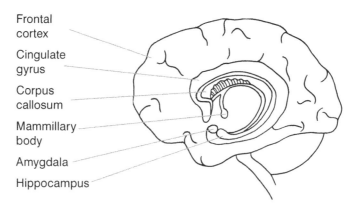

FIGURE 8.2. Brain anatomy and emotion.

instincts and mood; it is sometimes called the "old brain." Some parts of the limbic system are these:

- The hippocampus, involved in memory and learning.
- The amygdala, involved in automatic emotional responses to things in the world (e.g., a fearful or angry response to a noise in the middle of the night).
- The hypothalamus, a region involved in controlling hormones that regulate our responses to things in the world (e.g., releasing adrenaline to increase blood flow to our muscles, in preparation for a flight-or-fight response to the thought that a burglar may be breaking into our home).
- The insular cortex, which is involved in our awareness of body sensations linked to emotions (e.g., noticing our heartbeat speed up as we become scared at the thought of a burglary).
- The frontal neocortex, sometimes called the "new brain," allows us to weigh the similarities and differences between situations and to recognize the likely consequences of the actions we may take. It allows us to reason logically about what is going on and what we should do (e.g., how best to respond to the noise in the night) and can suppress emotional responses if necessary (e.g., reducing the tension when we realize the noise was not caused by a burglar).

The brain has two routes to emotional experience. The first—or "fast"—route goes straight from the sensory input to the amygdala in the limbic system and results in an immediate and strong emotional reaction. This is a primitive reaction and can save us from immediate harm or threat. For example, if a person were walking in the woods and suddenly a bear appeared in the path, reared up, and growled, that person would experience a strong fear response and an adrenaline boost to allow him or her to flee as quickly as possible. There would be no time for reasoning or logic. The second—or "slow"—route is via the frontal lobes and the hippocampus. These abilities allow us to weigh the dangers, consider alternative responses, compare the present situation to our experiences in the past, and choose the best response. This route combines the emotional response with a logical assessment of the situation, so that we can choose from several possible responses.

A brain injury can disrupt the delicate circuitry linking the frontal lobes with the limbic system. Damage either directly to the frontal lobes or to the connecting circuitry can lead to problems with emotional and behavioral control. The fast, instinctive, "old-brain" response can kick in right away, even in response to relatively minor stressors, resulting in experiences of strong emotions. The threat system may become overactive. Survivors of brain injury may feel that they are not in control of their emotions, but rather that their emotions are controlling them.

MAKING THE LINKS

Survivors of brain injury can face many difficult situations likely to have an emotional impact. Acquired impairments can affect everyday activities, causing repeated failure experiences (e.g., burning food by forgetting to take it out of the oven, due to impaired attention) or necessitating unwanted adaptations to their lives (e.g., modifying activities and housing to accommodate a change in mobility). There may be difficult medical aspects of their situation to manage, such as seizures, hormonal changes, sleep disorder, fatigue, sexual dysfunction, and medication side effects. Social roles and relationships may be adversely affected by the injury and its consequences. Survivors may have to take an extended period off work or be unable to return to work at all. Close relationships can be put under strain by the trauma of brain injury and the difficulties posed by its consequences—and, sadly, some relationships fail.

With all these challenging aspects of their situation, survivors of brain injury can lose self-esteem and become underoccupied and socially isolated. The combination of multiple difficult circumstances can lead to a sense of frustration or helplessness, which may act as a trigger for depression or anxiety disorders.

COMMON PRESENTING PROBLEMS

The following examples illustrate common difficulties reported by clients after brain injury:

- "I started to become really depressed when I kept making mistakes at work and got into trouble with my manager, who didn't understand."
- "I had so many problems managing everyday life that I was afraid I couldn't be the husband and dad I had been before my injury. I began to beat myself up a lot."
- "I became so scared the headaches meant I might have another bleed that sometimes I couldn't concentrate on anything else."
- "Now I have a really short fuse and can explode at the family at the smallest thing."

EXPLORING EMOTION AND EMOTIONAL PROBLEMS WITH CLIENTS

Having the opportunity to learn about how emotions can be affected by ABI—and even just being listened to—can sometimes provoke strong emotions in clients. If you are working in a group setting, it is important to have two people facilitating the group, so that if clients become distressed they have the option to leave the group with support for a break before returning. If group members are also having individual psychotherapy, it is important for the group facilitators and the psychotherapist to seek consent from these clients to share information before the group sessions begin, so that issues raised during the group can be explored further in psychotherapy.

Whether you are working with a group or on a one-to-one basis, allow plenty of time to expand on the materials and to support clients in relating the information to themselves. Be ready to provide examples to illustrate the educational material, such as the example of different responses to noises in the dark to illustrate how our interpretations of a situation influence our emotions. You may also need to illustrate the difference between vital, life-preserving, fast-track emotional responses (such as a threat response to the danger of seeing a bear in the woods, or a disgust response to prevent us from eating spoiled food) and similarly rapid responses to lesser threats (such as being stuck in traffic). It is best not to give examples from your own life and to stick to examples that are not extreme. Never push clients to give examples if they are reluctant to do so.

To start clients thinking about their own emotional responses, and to introduce the CBT cycle of thoughts–feelings–sensations–actions in a relatively unthreatening way, ask the clients, "How would you feel if you were walking down the street, and someone you know passes by and does not say hello?" Most people say they would feel angry, or hurt, or upset. Then ask the clients to consider whether they would notice any physical sensations surrounding these feelings (e.g., feeling themselves flush, becoming tearful, experiencing an increase in heart rate, feeling sick). Ask also how they would behave (e.g., avoiding or ignoring the person later, becoming angry toward the person).

Next, tell the clients that the person had sun in his or her eyes and could not see. Then ask how they would feel, given this new information. Have a discussion about how our immediate emotional reactions can be changed by the presence of additional information about the situation. Ask the clients to think of other examples where an emotional reaction might change when new information is given. One example would be a situation where someone pushes into the line at the cash register in a shop. Gather a first response to this situation; then add that the person has a sick child waiting in the car, and ask whether that information would change their emotional response.

The Brain and Emotion

Once clients have started to consider their own mood difficulties, it can be helpful to provide some more education about how the brain controls emotions. Handout 8.5 illustrates the distinction between the "old brain" (the limbic system and associated flight-or-fight responses) and the "new brain" (the frontal neocortex, which can make use of memory to generate reasoned responses based on past experience). You could expand on this by discussing the advantages and disadvantages of "old-brain" versus "new-brain" responses to different situations, such as facing a dental procedure (to run or to stay and have the procedure) or hearing someone walking behind you up a dark alleyway (to get away quickly or to spend time thinking about the situation).

As noted earlier, Handout 8.3 explains the three emotional systems (the threat, drive, and soothing systems). Role-play activity can be used to explore this further. Ask the clients to imagine that they are in a café and have been waiting to be served for ages. It is busy, crowded, and loud, and someone pushes in front to try to get served first. Ask them to act out what would happen if they had an "old-brain"/threat system response:

- What would a "fight" response look like?
- What would a "flight" response look like?
- What would a "freeze" response look like?

What Can Happen after Brain Injury?

Handout 8.6 focuses on common emotional difficulties after brain injury. Ask clients whether any of the problems listed in this handout (all described by people with ABI) resonate with them. Refer back to Handout 8.4 to explore some of the reasons why these problems occur after neurological damage (e.g., changes in regulation of emotion and behavior following damage to circuitry linking the frontal lobes with the limbic system).

Recording and Reflecting on Emotions and Coping Styles

Ask your clients to complete the 7-day mood diary provided as Handout 8.7. They should record any instances of difficult emotions (e.g., feeling sad, angry, or anxious) and, if possible, the situation in which the feelings occurred. Some clients with reduced awareness may need support to complete this diary. Review the clients' diaries with them to identify whether any particular mood difficulties happen more often than others, and whether there are any patterns in the situations involved. Support them as they consider how they felt physically as well as emotionally in these situations.

Now discuss with clients the relationships among thoughts, feelings, and behavior, using the CBT cycle illustrated in Handout 8.1. Encourage them to consider their mood diaries in the light of this cycle, and to develop their reflections accordingly. Discuss whether they were able to identify thoughts, feelings, and behaviors, and if not, what made this hard to do. You can make it easier by brainstorming lists of common feelings and physical sensations. A related group activity might be to think of a hypothetical situation (e.g., going to a party) and ask members to come up with different cycles of thoughts, feelings, physical sensations, and behaviors that someone at the party might have, depending on which emotional system is engaged. For instance, the person's threat system might be engaged by overhearing negative gossip about him or her, the drive system by wanting to talk to someone in particular, or the soothing system by being surrounded by good friends.

Once clients have learned about different types of emotional responses, and have started to think about their own responses, it can be helpful to consider coping styles commonly used in response to threats or stressful situations. Clients can complete a version of the Coping Inventory for Stressful Situations modified for people with ABI (Simblett, Gracey, Ring, & Bateman, 2015), to learn more about the kinds of coping strategies they use most naturally. It may also be helpful for clients to spend some time considering the strategies they used prior to their injury, and to think about whether these are still effective. Handout 8.8 can assist clients in thinking about all these things.

Next, consider with clients how the neurological damage caused by brain injury can affect coping responses. Coping can be challenging to begin with, as there are often new and difficult situations to deal with after brain injury, and brain injury itself can complicate coping efforts. Communication difficulties can make it harder to get social support. Cognitive impairments such as reduced processing speed, increased impulsivity/disinhibition, or impaired planning can affect task-focused coping. The strategies discussed by Winegardner in Chapter 5 of this workbook, such as increasing awareness in the moment (e.g., by using

Stop/Think), learning to anticipate difficulties, or planning what to do (e.g., by using the Goal Management Framework or GMF), may help.

REHABILITATION STRATEGIES

It is important to make sure you have enough time to introduce and demonstrate these strategies (at least 20–30 minutes for each one). Invite discussion of any concerns before starting to lead an exercise. To reduce any anxieties, cover what to do if an exercise does not seem to be working out (e.g., if a client in a group is having major difficulty, give permission for the client to stop the exercise and to sit quietly waiting for the others to finish). Explain that not all strategies are for everyone, and that this is why we introduce a number of different options that can be tried out. Emphasize that it is important to practice the strategies before using them in tough situations. Here is some advice you may wish to share with clients:

- Go at your own pace.
- Be kind to yourself.
- Using strategies needs practice, just like other skills you have developed, such as swimming or cycling.
- It is better to practice strategies either in therapy or alone when things are feeling OK, before trying them out when in an emotional state.
- Practicing strategies is easier on some days than on others.
- Practice makes using strategies easier.
- It is easier to learn to swim in the shallow end of a pool before jumping off into the deep end!

Using Compassion

"Compassion" means being sensitive to suffering in oneself and others, and being committed to trying to relieve this suffering. It includes these aspects:

- Kindness to ourselves and others, not judging.
- Acceptance—being open to feelings and tolerating them.
- Wisdom—knowing that we are not to blame, since we did not choose things to be as they are.
- Courage to do something to improve the situation.

Developing compassion toward ourselves can help to balance the three emotional systems, so we can be appropriately anxious, angry, excited, gentle, or kind when we need to be. We can use exercises such as mindfulness and compassionate imagery to develop our compassion.

Mindfulness

Being "mindful" means being fully in contact with our present experience, including both external events and our internal responses. If we are more aware of our thoughts, emotions, and physical sensations, we can react more objectively and less automatically. Mindfulness-based interventions have been found to be effective treatments for reducing symptoms of depression (Strauss, Cavanagh, Oliver, & Pettman, 2014), and there is promising evidence that they may reduce fatigue after stroke or brain injury (Johansson, Bjuhr, & Rönnbäck, 2012) and reduce symptoms of posttraumatic stress in the context of mild TBI (Cole et al., 2015).

Handout 8.9 provides some guidance on mindfulness for clients. Instructions for "compassionate mind" training exercises are available at the Compassionate Mind Foundation's website (*https.compassionatemind.co.uk*).

Calming Breaths

The "calming breaths" exercise can be helpful for halting the sensations of anxiety and panic when they begin to emerge, and can help achieve a deep state of relaxation quickly. You may want to use the script provided in Handout 8.10 with clients; they can also take it home to continue practicing with family members, friends, or caregivers.

Compassionate Imagery

Compassionate imagery is designed to stimulate the soothing system. Depending on the exercise used, clients can develop images of being in a safe place, or being with a compassionate person, or being compassionate themselves. For example, one client developed an image of feeling safe walking along the sand of a beautiful beach. Another client developed an image of a compassionate person in the client's family and would imagine that person's response to the difficulties the client was facing. It is also possible to develop an image of oneself becoming compassionate by imagining taking on the persona of a compassionate person. What would that person look and sound like? How would that person respond to different situations? Information for clients about compassionate imagery techniques is provided in Handout 8.11.

Progressive Muscle Relaxation

Progressive muscle relaxation is a technique to help people develop an awareness of muscular tension and an ability to release this tension to promote relaxation. A script is provided in Handout 8.12 for clients to use either in sessions or at home. It can be helpful to make an audio recording of this script so that it can be used at any time.

Cognitive Restructuring

A good time to introduce the CBT strategy of cognitive restructuring can be after reviewing the homework of monitoring thoughts and feelings. Thoughts that affect us negatively often ignore some of the facts or can be all-or-nothing (e.g., "I am 100% no good"). They can involve assuming the worst, also known as "catastrophizing" (e.g., "My husband is 10 minutes late home from work; he must have had a terrible accident"). Negative thoughts can pop up automatically, leading us to feel bad.

We can train ourselves to notice these thoughts and to examine the evidence for them. What were your clients thinking just before they felt angry, scared, or sad (e.g., "I'm useless, I can't do anything!")? Ask them to find evidence both supporting that thought (e.g., "I haven't managed to do what I planned to do today") and refuting it (e.g., "Maybe I'm fatigued because of my stroke, and that's making things hard today"). The next step is to come up with a new, balanced thought that takes all of the evidence into account (e.g., "I am making more mistakes than before because of my brain injury, but I often do things fine, especially when I use strategies to help me—I'll use fatigue management strategies tomorrow"). It can be helpful for clients to use copies of Handout 8.13 to record these events, and to keep them to refer to if a similar situation arises in the future. The written evidence of having reframed thoughts before can build self-efficacy and support the process of change when clients may be highly self-critical or unable to recall previous successes.

Behavioral Experiments

Acquired cognitive difficulties can make it difficult for clients to weigh evidence for and against beliefs in the abstract. When such difficulties are present, the CBT technique of behavioral experiments can be very helpful in providing real-world examples. Behavioral experiments use carefully planned experiential activities to help people gather information to test their existing beliefs and construct new, helpful beliefs (Bennett-Levy et al., 2004). For example, clients who fear that they will not be able to hold a social conversation after brain injury can be helped to carry out a behavioral experiment to find out whether the evidence supports this negative prediction, or an alternative prediction that they can talk with others, possibly with the help of relevant strategies (e.g., strategies to manage anxiety or communication difficulties). Not only do experiential activities provide concrete examples to discuss and reflect upon together, but the personal experience involved is likely to enhance learning (Bennett-Levy et al., 2004). An example of this comes from one of the case studies presented at the end of this chapter: David was supported in using an opportunity to present a news item at a community meeting as a behavioral experiment. He was guided to identify predictions about his ability to present the news item beforehand ("I will have word-finding difficulties and freeze when I am put on the spot" vs. "I may feel nervous and need to use strategies to manage the situation, but I will do OK"). He then carried out the task and was supported in reflecting upon his experience and feedback from others about his news item. This provided a powerful example of his ability to manage communicating to groups under pressure with the use of strategies. A template for planning behavioral experiments is provided in this workbook as Handout 5.12 (see Winegardner, Chapter 5).

Strategies to Boost Drive, Including Behavioral Activation

When clients become depressed or isolated, they tend to do less and less. This means that they become even more depressed, as they are not gaining enough reward through activity.

Supporting clients to become more active, to notice which activities they find most enjoyable or satisfying and to schedule these into each day, can help improve mood by boosting the drive system. This technique is called Behavioral Activation or Activity Scheduling.

Another way to help clients boost the drive system can be to encourage them to keep a "success log," to remember all the things that they have done well or that are positive. When we are depressed or preoccupied with anxiety or anger, we can forget the things that are going well!

You may also wish to refer to the section on emotional/behavioral regulation in Chapter 5 by Winegardner.

BRINGING IT ALL TOGETHER

As a final activity, you can ask clients to share something that helps them tackle the challenges facing them with courage. They can share this either with an individual therapist, with group facilitators and members, or with friends/family members. This could be something linked to a valued activity or role (e.g., something from a volunteer job they are doing or a club they belong to), or it could be linked to people who support them (e.g., a picture by one of their children or a photograph of a family member or pet). Some clients may wish to include pieces of writing, quotes, or music that they find inspiring or comforting.

COMPLETING A MOOD PROFILE

Help clients to draw together what they have learned about their emotional responses after brain injury and the coping strategies that work best for them by completing Handout 8.14 for their portfolios.

CASE STUDIES

It is important to note that mood difficulties can present very differently in clients with brain injury. Although Jeff (described in several earlier chapters), who sustained a very severe injury, definitely experienced frustration and loneliness, his limited awareness meant that he did not appear to experience a significant sense of felt distress. The problems Jeff faced in dealing with his postinjury emotions, and some of his goals and strategies for dealing with these problems, are described in Table 8.1.

By contrast, another client, David, was extremely aware of and distressed by the changes he faced after a mild TBI. David was knocked off his bike at the age of 52. He was given the "all-clear" at his local emergency room; however, he experienced ongoing symptoms, including severe headaches, fatigue, mood disturbance, and cognitive difficulties. David was eventually given a diagnosis of severe postconcussion syndrome. Table 8.2 describes the problems David faced in dealing with his postinjury mood issues, and some of his goals and strategies for dealing with these.

TABLE 8.1. Dealing with Jeff's Mood-Related Challenges

Challenges	Goals and strategies	Context for rehabilitation
Low mood, loss of confidence, loneliness, irritability, frustration, aggressive verbal outbursts Jeff sometimes drank too much as a way of coping with his feelings. This made his irritability even worse, affecting relationships with family members and leading to increased loneliness and isolation. *Loss of planned future* As noted in earlier chapters, Jeff had been a promising golfer as a teenager, and had been planning to take up a sports scholarship in the United States prior to his injury. After the accident, he watched as his friends and siblings moved on, building careers and relationships, leaving him behind. The changes in him after brain injury made it even harder for him to maintain social relationships.	Goals: To increase self-confidence, and reduce irritability/low mood in order to improve family relationships and friendships. Strategies: • Positive psychology approaches to strengthen sense of self and identity. • Behavioral experiments in a range of activities and contexts, to build confidence and trial strategies. • "Calming breaths" exercise to manage frustration and anger in the moment.	Mood work was incorporated into all of Jeff's project-based activities. Engaging once again in meaningful activities boosted his self-esteem by enhancing his feelings of pleasure and mastery and offering him opportunities to connect with others, reducing his loneliness.

TABLE 8.2. Dealing with David's Mood-Related Challenges

Challenges	Goals and strategies	Context for rehabilitation
Anxiety, anger, nightmares David had always had high standards for himself at work and at home. After his mild TBI, he found himself struggling to manage everyday tasks and became very critical of himself. He developed difficulties with anxiety, low mood, anger and nightmares, and found it harder to manage pressure at work. *Low mood, rumination, self-criticism* David frequently berated himself for struggling with previously simple tasks when his injury was relatively mild. *High expectations, sensitivity to even minor errors* David found himself trapped in a vicious cycle: His low mood meant that he struggled to use strategies and made even more minor errors; the increase in errors led to increased self-criticism and withdrawal from participation, further worsening his mood. *Irritability and short temper with his children* David's daughter asked, "When will I get my daddy back?" *Passive suicidality* David reported taking his dog for walks down dark back streets, in the hope that he would be mugged and killed	Goals: To understand his brain injury and use strategies to manage difficulties across different situations (e.g., at home with his wife and children and at work). Also, to reduce how often he had nightmares. Strategies: • David was offered trauma-focused CBT and CFT. • To reduce his anxiety about the chance of having nightmares, he used a breathing exercise before going to bed and spent time visualizing a safe place. • To reduce his self-criticism, he visualized a compassionate person and imagined what that person would say to him in various situations.	David engaged in a range of activities to support his return to work, all of which incorporated mood management strategies. David researched, planned, and presented a news item at a community meeting. He deliberately chose a contentious topic, as he knew that he would be challenged in meetings at work, and he needed to build confidence in a safe setting. By adopting strategies to reduce anxiety and develop a compassionate approach to himself, he found he could better manage tasks that had previously been difficult after his mild TBI. David used mood management strategies prior to engaging in problem-solving activities to minimize the intrusion of negative thoughts and self-critical ruminations, and to strengthen his ability to direct all of his attention to the problem at hand.

REFERENCES

Anderson, C. S., Linto, J., & Stewart-Wynne, E. G. (1995). A population-based assessment of the impact and burden of caregiving for long-term stroke survivors. *Stroke, 26*(5), 843–849.

Ashman, T., Cantor, J. B., Tsaousides, T., Spielman, L., & Gordon, W. (2014). Comparison of cognitive behavioral therapy and supportive psychotherapy for the treatment of depression following traumatic brain injury: A randomized controlled trial. *Journal of Head Trauma Rehabilitation, 29*(6), 467–478.

Ashworth, F., Clarke, A., Jones, L., Jennings, C., & Longworth, C. (2015). An exploration of compassion focused therapy following acquired brain injury. *Psychology and Psychotherapy, 88*(2), 143–162.

Beck, A. T., Rush, A. J., Shaw, B. F., & Emery, G. (1979). *Cognitive therapy of depression.* New York: Guilford Press.

Bennett-Levy, J., Westbrook, D., Fennell, M., Cooper, M., Rouf, K., & Hackmann, A. (2004). Behavioural experiments: Historical and conceptual underpinnings. In J. Bennett-Levy, D. Westbrook, M. Fennell, M. Cooper, K. Rouf, & A. Hackmann (Eds.), *Oxford guide to behavioural experiments in cognitive therapy* (pp. 1–20). Oxford, UK: Oxford University Press.

Bowen, A., Chamberlain, M. A., Tennant, A., Neumann, V., & Conner, M. (1999). The persistence of mood disorders following traumatic brain injury: A 1-year follow-up. *Brain Injury, 13*(7), 547–553.

Broomfield, N. M., Laidlaw, K., Hickabottom, E., Murray, M. F., Pendrey, R., Whittick, J. E., & Gillespie, D. C. (2011). Post-stroke depression: The case for augmented, individually tailored cognitive behavioural therapy. *Clinical Psychology and Psychotherapy, 18*(3), 202–217.

Cole, M. A., Muir, J. J., Gans, J. J., Shin, L. M., D'Esposito, M., Harel, B. T., & Schembri, A. (2015). Simultaneous treatment of neurocognitive and psychiatric symptoms in veterans with post-traumatic stress disorder and history of mild traumatic brain injury: A pilot study of mindfulness-based stress reduction. *Military Medicine, 180*(9), 956–963.

Dewar, B. K., & Gracey, F. (2007). 'Am not was': Cognitive-behavioural therapy for adjustment and identity change following herpes simplex encephalitis. *Neuropsychological Rehabilitation, 17*(4–5), 602–620.

Evans, J. J. (2011). Positive psychology and brain injury rehabilitation. *Brain Impairment, 12*(2), 117–127.

Fann, J. R., Bombardier, C. H., Vannoy, S., Dyer, J., Ludman, E., Dikmen, S., . . . Temkin, N. (2015). Telephone and in-person cognitive behavioral therapy for major depression after traumatic brain injury: A randomized controlled trial. *Journal of Neurotrauma, 32*(1), 45–57.

Gilbert, P. (2000). Social mentalities: Internal 'social' conflicts and the role of inner warmth and compassion in cognitive therapy. In P. Gilbert & K. G. Bailey (Eds.), *Genes on the couch: Explorations in evolutionary psychotherapy* (pp. 118–150). Hove, UK: Brunner–Routledge.

Gilbert, P. (2010a). *Compassion focused therapy: Distinctive features.* Hove, UK: Routledge.

Gilbert, P. (Ed.). (2010b). Compassion focused therapy [Special issue]. *International Journal of Cognitive Therapy, 3,* 95–210.

Gracey, F., Oldham, P., & Kritzinger, R. (2007). Finding out if 'The "me" will shut down': Successful cognitive-behavioural therapy of seizure-related panic symptoms following subarachnoid haemorrhage. A single case report. *Neuropsychological Rehabilitation, 17*(1), 106–119.

Greenberger, D., & Padesky, C. A. (2015). *Mind over mood: Change how you feel by changing the way you think* (2nd ed.). New York: Guilford Press.

Hackett, M. L., & Pickles, K. (2014). Part I: Frequency of depression after stroke: An updated systematic review and meta-analysis of observational studies. *International Journal of Stroke, 9*(8), 1017–1025.

Hibbard, M. R., Uysal, S., Kepler, K., Bogdany, J., & Silver, J. (1998). Axis II psychopathology in individuals with traumatic brain injury. *Journal of Head Trauma Rehabilitation, 13,* 24–39.

House, A., Knapp, P., Bamford, J., & Vail, A. (2001). Mortality at 12 and 24 months after stroke may be associated with depressive symptoms at 1 month. *Stroke, 32*(3), 696–701.

Johansson, B., Bjuhr, H., & Rönnbäck, L. (2012). Mindfulness-based stress reduction (MBSR) improves long-term mental fatigue after stroke or traumatic brain injury. *Brain Injury, 26*, 1–8.

Lazarus, R. R. S., & Folkman, S. (1987). Transactional theory and research on emotions and coping. *European Journal of Personality, 1*, 141–169.

Lincoln, N. B., & Flannaghan, T. (2003). Cognitive behavioral psychotherapy for depression following stroke: A randomized controlled trial. *Stroke, 34*(1), 111–115.

Malia, K., Powell, G., & Torode, S. (1995). Coping and psychosocial function after brain injury. *Brain Injury, 9*(6), 607–618.

Moore, A. D., & Stambrook, M. (1992). Coping strategies and locus of control following traumatic brain injury: Relationship to long-term outcome. *Brain Injury, 6*(1), 89–94.

NHS Improvement—Stroke. (2011). *Psychological care after stroke: Improving stroke services for people with cognitive and mood disorders.* Leicester, UK: NHS Improvement. Retrieved from *www.nice.org.uk/media/default/sharedlearning/531_strokepsychologicalsupportfinal.pdf.*

Parikh, R. M., Robinson, R. G., Lipsey, J. R., Starkstein, S. E., Fedoroff, J. P., & Price, T. R. (1990). The impact of poststroke depression on recovery in activities of daily living over a 2-year follow-up. *Archives of Neurology, 47*(7), 785–789.

Pohjasvaara, T., Vataja, R., Leppävuori, A., Kaste, M., & Erkinjuntti, T. (2001). Depression is an independent predictor of poor long-term functional outcome post-stroke. *European Journal of Neurology, 8*(4), 315–319.

Seligman, M. E. P. (2002). *Authentic happiness: Using the new positive psychology to realize your potential for lasting fulfillment.* New York: Free Press.

Seligman, M. E. P., Steen, T. A., Park, N., & Peterson, C. (2005). Positive psychology progress: Empirical validation of interventions. *American Psychologist, 60*(5), 410–421.

Simblett, S. K., Gracey, F., Ring, H., & Bateman, A. (2015). Measuring coping style following acquired brain injury: A modification of the Coping Inventory for Stressful Situations using Rasch analysis. *British Journal of Clinical Psychology, 54*(3), 249–265.

Sinyor, D., Amato, P., Kaloupek, D. G., Becker, R., Goldenberg, M., & Coopersmith, H. (1986). Post-stroke depression: Relationships to functional impairment, coping strategies, and rehabilitation outcome. *Stroke, 17*(6), 1102–1107.

Strauss, C., Cavanagh, K., Oliver, A., & Pettman, D. (2014). Mindfulness-based interventions for people diagnosed with a current episode of an anxiety or depressive disorder: A meta-analysis of randomised controlled trials. *PLoS ONE, 9*(4), 1–13.

Waldron, B., Casserly, L. M., & O'Sullivan, C. (2013). Cognitive behavioural therapy for depression and anxiety in adults with acquired brain injury: What works for whom? *Neuropsychological Rehabilitation, 23*(1), 64–101.

The Cognitive-Behavioral Therapy (CBT) Cycle

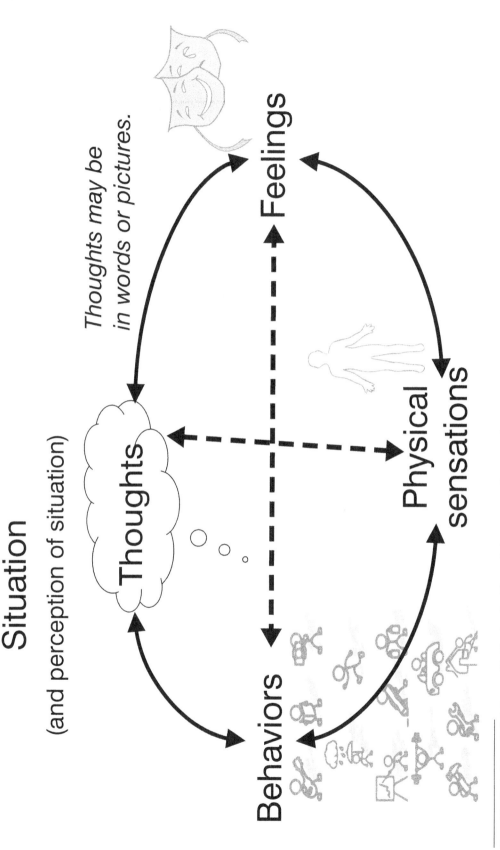

Situation
(and perception of situation)

Thoughts may be in words or pictures.

Thoughts

Feelings

Physical sensations

Behaviors

From *The Brain Injury Rehabilitation Workbook*, edited by Rachel Winson, Barbara A. Wilson, and Andrew Bateman. Copyright © 2017 The Guilford Press. Permission to photocopy this handout is granted to purchasers of this book for personal use or for use with individual clients (see copyright page for details). Purchasers can download additional copies of this handout (see the box at the end of the table of contents).

Thinking, Feeling, Doing

Physical Sensations

- Physical sensations can warn us that the threat system has been activated. We can learn to notice this.
- Some things to look out for:
  - Heart racing.
  - Feeling hot, face getting red.
  - Clenched fists, tense muscles.

Behavior

- An active threat system can influence our behavior.
- Some things to look out for:
  - The "fight" response—showing anger toward others.
  - The "flight" response—avoiding or leaving situations.
  - The "freeze" response—shutting down.

Thoughts and Feelings

- Our thoughts and emotions can often activate the threat system (e.g., "What if I fall?", "How dare they treat me as if I'm stupid?", "Why on earth did I make the same mistake again?").

From *The Brain Injury Rehabilitation Workbook*, edited by Rachel Winson, Barbara A. Wilson, and Andrew Bateman. Copyright © 2017 The Guilford Press. Permission to photocopy this handout is granted to purchasers of this book for personal use or for use with individual clients (see copyright page for details). Purchasers can download additional copies of this handout (see the box at the end of the table of contents).

Three Emotion Systems

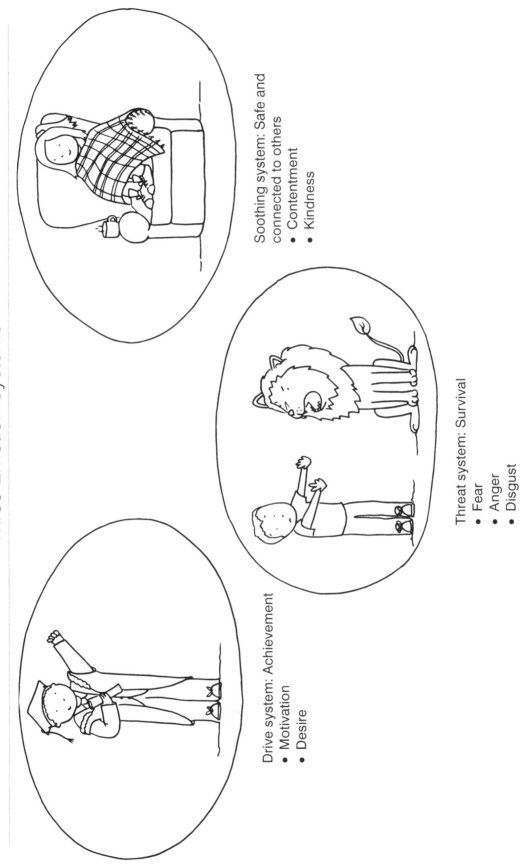

Drive system: Achievement
- Motivation
- Desire

Threat system: Survival
- Fear
- Anger
- Disgust

Soothing system: Safe and connected to others
- Contentment
- Kindness

From *The Brain Injury Rehabilitation Workbook*, edited by Rachel Winson, Barbara A. Wilson, and Andrew Bateman. Copyright © 2017 The Guilford Press. Permission to photocopy this handout is granted to purchasers of this book for personal use or for use with individual clients (see copyright page for details). Purchasers can download additional copies of this handout (see the box at the end of the table of contents).

Brain Anatomy and Emotion

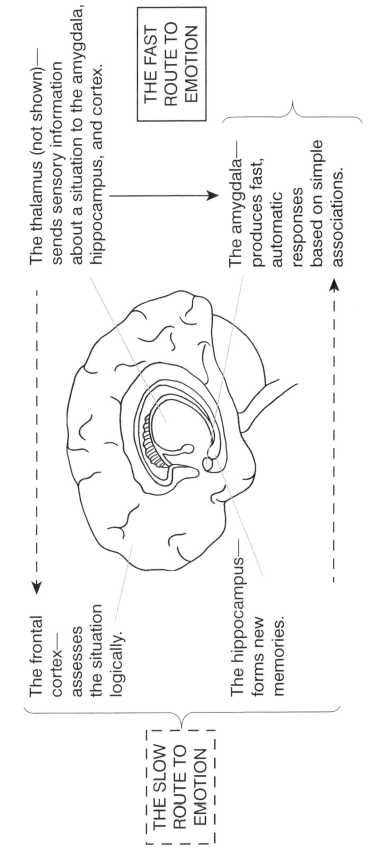

THE FAST ROUTE TO EMOTION

The thalamus (not shown)—sends sensory information about a situation to the amygdala, hippocampus, and cortex.

The amygdala—produces fast, automatic responses based on simple associations.

The frontal cortex—assesses the situation logically.

The hippocampus—forms new memories.

THE SLOW ROUTE TO EMOTION

From *The Brain Injury Rehabilitation Workbook*, edited by Rachel Winson, Barbara A. Wilson, and Andrew Bateman. Copyright © 2017 The Guilford Press. Permission to photocopy this handout is granted to purchasers of this book for personal use or for use with individual clients (see copyright page for details). Purchasers can download additional copies of this handout (see the box at the end of the table of contents).

Understanding Emotions: New Brain/Old Brain

- There are primitive parts of our brain, deep inside, that we share with other animals. We refer to these parts as the "old brain."
- The "old brain" produces automatic emotional responses like anger, fear, or disgust when we encounter a threat.
- It also produces our feelings of lust.
- These responses are natural and help us to survive and reproduce.

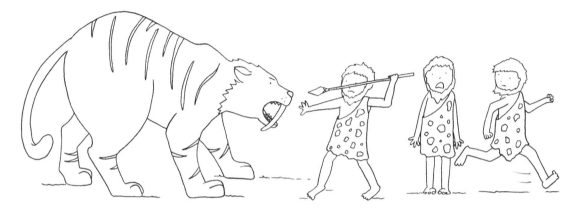

- The "new brain" is more sophisticated. It helps us with:
  - Reasoning.
  - Imagining.
  - Making decisions and planning.
  - Being aware of ourselves.
- It can also help keep "old-brain" responses under control!

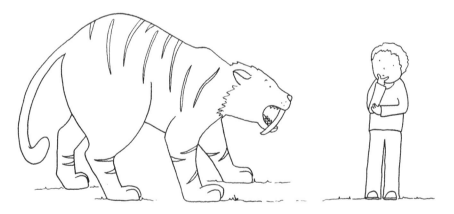

- A brain injury can:
  - Damage parts of the "new brain."
  - Disrupt connections between the "new brain" and "old brain."

From *The Brain Injury Rehabilitation Workbook*, edited by Rachel Winson, Barbara A. Wilson, and Andrew Bateman. Copyright © 2017 The Guilford Press. Permission to photocopy this handout is granted to purchasers of this book for personal use or for use with individual clients (see copyright page for details). Purchasers can download additional copies of this handout (see the box at the end of the table of contents).

Do You Ever . . . ?

Thoughts

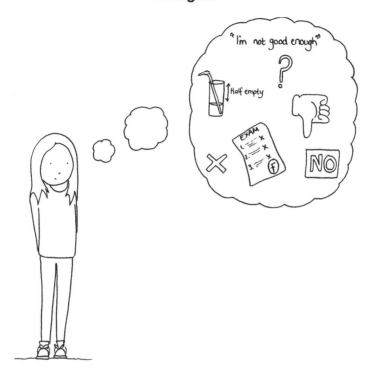

- Is it harder now to stop thoughts you don't want (ruminating)?
- Do you have trouble reflecting on whether a thought is accurate?

Emotions

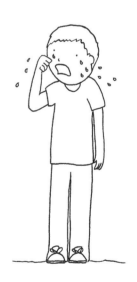

- Do you get irritated more easily?
- Do you cry for no good reason?
- Do you laugh when you shouldn't?
- Does it feel like your emotions are closer to the surface? Do your emotions control you, rather than your controlling them?

(continued)

From *The Brain Injury Rehabilitation Workbook*, edited by Rachel Winson, Barbara A. Wilson, and Andrew Bateman. Copyright © 2017 The Guilford Press. Permission to photocopy this handout is granted to purchasers of this book for personal use or for use with individual clients (see copyright page for details). Purchasers can download additional copies of this handout (see the box at the end of the table of contents).

Words and Actions

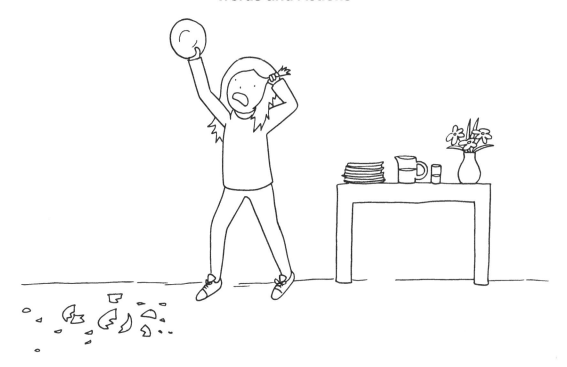

- Do you ever say things you never intended to say?
- Do you ever do things you wish you hadn't?
- Do you react to things more quickly than before, as if the brakes had suddenly come off?
- Do you ever yell or throw things when you never wanted to?

Mood Diary

Date and time	Situation: What was happening?	How did I feel?	What was I thinking at the time?	How did my body feel at the time?	What did I do?

From *The Brain Injury Rehabilitation Workbook*, edited by Rachel Winson, Barbara A. Wilson, and Andrew Bateman. Copyright © 2017 The Guilford Press. Permission to photocopy this handout is granted to purchasers of this book for personal use or for use with individual clients (see copyright page for details). Purchasers can download additional copies of this handout (see the box at the end of the table of contents).

How Do You Cope?

- How did you tend to cope with difficulties in life before your brain injury (e.g., through problem solving, getting support from others, distracting yourself from the problem)?

- How have you coped with difficulties since your brain injury?

- Can you think of examples when you coped well with the brain injury?

- What kind of skills do you think you have to enable you to cope effectively?

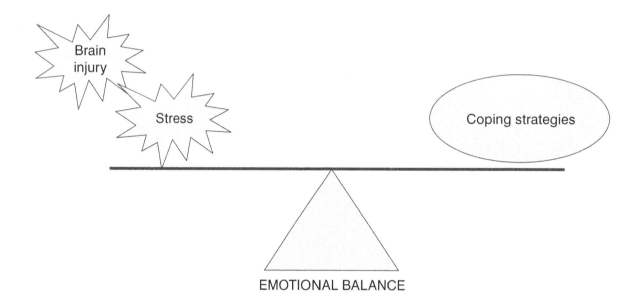

From *The Brain Injury Rehabilitation Workbook*, edited by Rachel Winson, Barbara A. Wilson, and Andrew Bateman. Copyright © 2017 The Guilford Press. Permission to photocopy this handout is granted to purchasers of this book for personal use or for use with individual clients (see copyright page for details). Purchasers can download additional copies of this handout (see the box at the end of the table of contents).

Mindfulness

- Mindfulness is paying attention to the present moment without judgment.

- Mindfulness involves observing our thoughts and feelings as they come up, and accepting and working with them.

- The skill of mindfulness is noticing when our minds wander and where they have wandered to, and then gently bringing them back to our focus. It is not about "getting it right"!

- Mindfulness can help us to notice and stand back. It can help to endure the discomfort of not acting on certain emotions, such as anger, irritability, anxiety, or distress.

- Try focusing gently on your breath going in and out, noticing if your attention wanders, and bringing it back to your breath without judgment.

- Or try focusing on eating a chocolate—first paying attention to how it looks and smells, and then slowly noticing how it feels to eat it and how it tastes.

From *The Brain Injury Rehabilitation Workbook*, edited by Rachel Winson, Barbara A. Wilson, and Andrew Bateman. Copyright © 2017 The Guilford Press. Permission to photocopy this handout is granted to purchasers of this book for personal use or for use with individual clients (see copyright page for details). Purchasers can download additional copies of this handout (see the box at the end of the table of contents).

Calming Breaths

- Breathing from your abdomen, inhale slowly as you count up to 5.

- Pause and hold your breath to a count of 5.

- Exhale slowly, through your nose or mouth, to a count of 5. Be sure to exhale fully.

- Now take two normal breaths.

- Keep up this exercise for about 5 minutes, going through the steps above about 10 times. If you feel lightheaded at any stage, stop for 30 seconds and then try again.

- Throughout the exercise, keep your breathing smooth and regular, without gulping in breaths or breathing out suddenly.

- You may also want to try saying a calming word every time you exhale—for example, "Calm," "Let go," or "Relax."

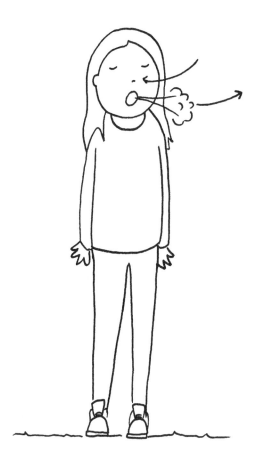

From *The Brain Injury Rehabilitation Workbook*, edited by Rachel Winson, Barbara A. Wilson, and Andrew Bateman. Copyright © 2017 The Guilford Press. Permission to photocopy this handout is granted to purchasers of this book for personal use or for use with individual clients (see copyright page for details). Purchasers can download additional copies of this handout (see the box at the end of the table of contents).

Compassionate Imagery

Compassion is:

- *Kindness* to ourselves and others, not judging.
- *Acceptance*—being open to feelings and tolerating them.
- *Wisdom*—knowing that we are not to blame, since we did not choose things to be as they are.
- *Courage* to do something to improve the situation.

Here are three types of compassionate imagery for you to try. These techniques are from the Compassionate Mind Foundation and more details can be found on their website (*https://compassionatemind.co.uk*).

1. *Safe-place imagery.* Allow an image of somewhere you feel safe and accepted to come to mind (such as a beautiful beach, a sunlit clearing in the woods, or a comfortable chair by a log fire). Pay attention to how it looks, sounds, smells, and feels. Imagine that in this place you are welcome and accepted.

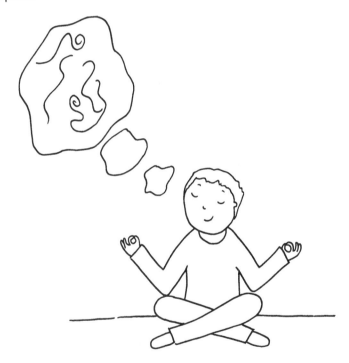

2. *A compassionate other.* Develop a mental image of someone who is perfectly compassionate toward you. (This can be either a real or an imaginary person.) What would this person look and sound like? What would the person say to you? What would it feel like to spend time with him or her?

3. *Becoming more compassionate.* Develop an image of yourself as someone who is truly compassionate. What would you look like? What would you do and say?

From *The Brain Injury Rehabilitation Workbook*, edited by Rachel Winson, Barbara A. Wilson, and Andrew Bateman. Copyright © 2017 The Guilford Press. Permission to photocopy this handout is granted to purchasers of this book for personal use or for use with individual clients (see copyright page for details). Purchasers can download additional copies of this handout (see the box at the end of the table of contents).

Progressive Muscle Relaxation

Choose a quiet, comfortable environment. Sit or lie down comfortably and close your eyes. Remember to breathe slowly and regularly during the exercise. If there are any movements you cannot make or which are uncomfortable or painful for you, please leave these movements out.

- Start with your feet. Pull your toes back; tense the muscles in your feet for about 5 seconds. Now relax the tension. And again pull your toes back; tense the muscles in your feet for about 5 seconds. Now relax the tension. Focus on how your feet feel when they are relaxed.

- Now straighten and tense your legs, pointing your toes, and hold this position for 5 seconds. Now relax and let your legs go limp. Now again straighten and tense your legs, pointing your toes, and hold the position. Relax again and let your legs go limp. Feel your muscles relaxing more and more deeply. Enjoy the feeling of relaxation.

- Next, tense your stomach muscles by pulling them in and up, as if you were preparing to receive a punch. Hold this position for about 5 seconds. Relax the tension. And again tense your stomach muscles. Relax the tension.

- Now arch your back, holding the tension for about 5 seconds. And relax. Again, arch your back and relax.

- Drop your head to your chest, and feel the tension in the back of your neck. Now lift your shoulders to your ears and hold the tension. Circle your shoulders around a couple of times, and then let them drop even further. Enjoy the feeling of your muscles relaxing more and more deeply.

- Now move on to your hands and arms. Stretch out your arms, making a tight fist with each hand. Hold the tension, then unclench your fists and relax your hands and arms. And again stretch out your arms and make tight fists. Hold, then relax.

- Concentrate on your face. Tense your forehead and jaw. Lower your eyebrows and bite hard, holding the tension. Now relax. Again, tense, hold the tension, and now relax.

- Finally, focus on your whole body. Tense your entire body. Your feet, legs, abdomen, back, shoulders and neck, arms, and face. Hold the tension for a few seconds. Now relax. And again tense your entire body, holding the tension for a few seconds. Now relax.

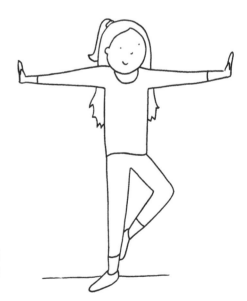

Feel your muscles relaxing more and more deeply. Your body is completely relaxed now. Enjoy the feeling. Think of what the relaxed feeling brings to your mind's eye, and notice any images or memories. Enjoy the whole of this relaxed feeling, and take a mental snapshot of it, so you can bring it to mind at other times.

Once you feel completely relaxed, count backward from 4 to 1. At 4, begin to feel more alert now; at 3, get ready to move again; at 2, start to become aware of your surroundings; at 1, open your eyes, feeling refreshed and relaxed. When you are ready, stand up slowly and stretch gently.

From *The Brain Injury Rehabilitation Workbook*, edited by Rachel Winson, Barbara A. Wilson, and Andrew Bateman. Copyright © 2017 The Guilford Press. Permission to photocopy this handout is granted to purchasers of this book for personal use or for use with individual clients (see copyright page for details). Purchasers can download additional copies of this handout (see the box at the end of the table of contents).

What's the Evidence?

- What were you thinking just before you felt angry, scared, or sad? (Example: "I'm useless! I can't do anything!")

- What evidence supports that thought? (Example: "I haven't managed to do what I planned to do today.")

- What evidence does not support that thought? What else might be going on? (Example: "Maybe I'm fatigued because of my stroke, and that's making things hard today.")

- What thought sums up all the evidence in a balanced way? (Example: "It's been a difficult day because I'm fatigued, so I will use fatigue management strategies tomorrow.")

From *The Brain Injury Rehabilitation Workbook*, edited by Rachel Winson, Barbara A. Wilson, and Andrew Bateman. Copyright © 2017 The Guilford Press. Permission to photocopy this handout is granted to purchasers of this book for personal use or for use with individual clients (see copyright page for details). Purchasers can download additional copies of this handout (see the box at the end of the table of contents).

My Mood Profile

Areas of the brain involved in emotion regulation that were affected by my brain injury include _____

_____

_____

_____

_____

Because of my injury, I sometimes find that I _____

_____

_____

_____

My ability to cope with difficulties is also influenced by _____

_____

_____

_____

The strategies I've found most helpful in managing these difficulties are _____

_____

_____

_____

_____

_____

_____

_____

_____

_____

_____

From *The Brain Injury Rehabilitation Workbook*, edited by Rachel Winson, Barbara A. Wilson, and Andrew Bateman. Copyright © 2017 The Guilford Press. Permission to photocopy this handout is granted to purchasers of this book for personal use or for use with individual clients (see copyright page for details). Purchasers can download additional copies of this handout (see the box at the end of the table of contents).

CHAPTER 9

Working with Identity Change after Brain Injury

Fergus Gracey
Leyla Prince
Rachel Winson

Identity is the glue that holds us together, joining a feeling of "being ourselves" in the present moment with the life experiences we have had in the past, and our sense of ourselves in the future. Within the holistic model of rehabilitation—and indeed, arguably, in any approach to rehabilitation that is concerned with the whole of human experience—identity should be a consideration in all aspects, not a stand-alone issue. This chapter has been placed toward the end of the book as a way of bringing together learning from all the areas previously covered. It is in the coming together of all our strengths and strategies to manage challenges in day-to-day living that our identities become real and open to experience.

WHAT IS IDENTITY?

The notion of "identity" is central to the field of psychology and has rightly received a great deal of attention from thinkers and researchers. As with many things in psychology, it is difficult to say exactly what identity "is." It is not something that can be measured with a ruler, looked at through a microscope, or brought into existence in a flash like subatomic particles in the Large Hadron Collider! However, it is something that, as humans, we all have a sense of. We can think of identity as a felt and experienced thing, which can be observed only within the mind's eye; nevertheless, identity can be talked about, and its essence can be shared with others.

Brain Systems and Identity

In recent years, neuroscientists have developed ideas about how certain brain systems can support what we experience as a sense of "self." Antonio Damasio (2000, 2005) and Joseph LeDoux (1998) are two pioneers in this growing field, called social and affective neuroscience. The brain areas associated with the self or identity include the functions that support our ability to remember multiple experiences throughout our lives, as well as systems that deal with our senses and internal experience of things (e.g., not only having a memory of an event, but reexperiencing the feelings we may have had at the time). These areas, including the frontal lobes and the hippocampi, are also vulnerable to the effects of brain injury.

Cognitive Systems and Identity

It is generally thought these days that we have multiple selves or identities, rather than a single, monolithic personality or identity (see Yeates, Gracey, & McGrath, 2008, for a review). Usually only one of these is in operation at any one time. For example, each of us may have a professional identity, and other identities that guide our actions in family or social situations. Each identity is rooted in a long string of experiences, so we can probably piece together a narrative that includes work history, relationships, and other interests.

We can also use these experiences to engage in "mental time travel" and imagine what kind of future we might have in these aspects of our lives. Martin Conway (2005) proposes a cognitive model of identity in which there is a "self-system" with two aspects:

1. A storage aspect that accrues all our lived experiences; categorizes these; and extracts patterns of meaning, feeling, and context that make up the various selves each of us can "be" at any given time.
2. An executive or goal management aspect that Conway calls "the working self." One self is active at a given time and sits on top of the executive system, helping to filter and focus motivation toward the goals and values that are most relevant to that particular self.

In Conway's model, then, our identity tries to make us more efficient in our day-to-day lives—helping our brains to predict and prioritize what's important, and to have certain patterns of behavior or interpretation online and ready to be activated in a relevant situation. When we want to think about the future or the past, we do so through the lens of a particular self, and this lends a sense of coherence and continuity to our moment-to-moment experience. When we recall experiences, certain facts and aspects of a situation may be excluded or altered so as to fit within the world view of that particular self. Conway (2005) provides an excellent account of the tension between coherence of memory (in terms of our own experiences) and correspondence of memory with reality. Although we all presume we have an accurate view of ourselves and the world, really this sense of coherence is a construction; we are all, to a greater or lesser extent, constructing a version of the world at each moment. This is an important idea, because it allows the idea of clients' difficulty in "owning" their various deficits after brain injury to be radically reinterpreted as an indication of the functioning self-system working hard to maintain coherence. It is very difficult for the brain to fit unanticipated and self-discrepant problems into a coherent sense of self.

Emotional Systems and Identity

The higher-order "self-system" sits on top of and is integrated with the lower-order "old brain" (see Ford, Chapter 8, this volume). Basically, the old brain or limbic system has the capacity to override the self-system under conditions of (perceived) threat, danger, or reward. However, the self-system also has the potential to filter our experiences so as to be biased toward seeing negatives or threats. Someone who has had a lot of negative life experiences will have developed a set of personal memories from which are extracted beliefs, feelings, and behaviors that make up a particular identity. This could mean that the person's self-system has developed so as to make it easier for the threat system to kick in, even when this is not actually needed. For example, in an ambiguous social situation, the system may default to presuming that there is a threat. So it is important to view such a person's current experiences and reactions as understandable, given the influence of past experiences.

Social Systems and Identity

Social psychologists look upon identity as rooted in social context. Our identities can be considered in terms of the roles we fulfill; the families, friendships, and activity groups we belong to; and what all these mean to us. Social identity theory proposes that we internalize these social identities (perhaps through our memories of experiences) and carry them as personal identities. Our social identities provide us with supports or resources we can draw upon. For example, we may draw on particular friendships for sympathy, practical advice, assistance, or distraction if we are facing a challenge or stress. Discussing a problem with friends can help identify new perspectives and solutions.

To summarize, identity is elusive. It can be thought of in terms of brain systems, processes of thinking and feeling, and social factors. But, really, it is just an idea that can help us try to make sense of our experiences; it is a set of beliefs about ourselves and predictions about how we will respond in certain situations, informed by recurring patterns in our life experiences. Our multiple selves are personally experienced, both in the moment in our day-to-day lives, and when we engage in mental time travel into past memories and future plans. The lens of identity through which we see the world can at times unconsciously twist things to give us a sense of coherence. We think that because of this combination of factors, the notion of "self" goes a long way toward helping make sense of people's experiences following brain injury. In fact, instead of focusing on medical diagnoses such as anxiety and depressive disorders, and working with (for instance) aggression or lack of insight as "problems," it may be more helpful to reconceptualize the challenges a client faces after brain injury as understandable aspects of a self-system struggling under the weight of multiple threats to social and personal identities. This can also provide a basis for thinking about some emerging ideas in brain injury rehabilitation—ideas having to do with positive experiences and identities, such as growth and the sense of joy, connectedness, ease, and freedom known in positive psychology as "flow" (Ownsworth, 2014).

HOW DOES BRAIN INJURY AFFECT IDENTITY?

As we have discussed, identity is personally experienced in the past, present, and future; it emerges from a mix of brain systems, psychological processes, and social groups and activities, any or all of which can be disrupted by brain injury. So it is very easy to understand why a proportion of people who have had a brain injury will experience a sense that their identities are under threat as their self-systems struggle with multiple challenges. Social and personal roles can be altered following brain injury. The self-system may also have reduced cognitive resources to help to update itself—so a client may be unable to recall either pre- or postinjury experiences that could contribute to a new or updated identity. Brain injury can also affect the system's ability to use a particular "working self" to inhibit the old brain/limbic system and regulate emotions and behavior. The threat to identity may manifest itself as anger, shame, embarrassment, worry, or denial of difficulties, as the brain's self-system seeks to reduce "in-the-moment" threat through various means.

All of these factors can be challenges for many clients, but especially for those who may have not been the most confident persons even prior to their injury, or for those whose self-worth is tied tightly to being highly effective in certain areas. In addition, because identity is based on massed experiences in the memory system, younger people have more fluid and less well-developed identities. Identity is thought to emerge during adolescence, and key self-defining autobiographical memories typically occur in late adolescence and early adulthood. This timing can create particular challenges for people who have sustained brain injury at younger ages. As one young man said, "How can I have any goals if I don't know who I am?" With younger people, work with family members and friendship groups may be especially important; the rehabilitation task here is to help the young persons to negotiate this stage of development successfully (Ylvisaker & Feeney, 2000). For many young people, the loss of friendships that can occur after brain injury robs them of the opportunity for the kinds of social experiences that are fundamental to identity development, so they become "stuck" in their development of identity.

Since identity starts in our felt sense of our day-to-day experiences, perhaps the best starting point is to think about how it might be affected by some of the specific experiences of life after a brain injury. Imagine that you're a senior executive in charge of multiple contracts for an international company. You are responsible for managing a large team, with a busy daily schedule of meetings, and you work long hours. You might describe yourself as a workaholic, ambitious, efficient, motivated. After brain injury, you need external aids to prompt you to do the simplest of daily tasks. You find it hard to explain yourself to your family and friends, let alone run work meetings about complex topics. And the fatigue you experience is so overwhelming that you have to rest for an hour after getting dressed in the morning. Or perhaps you're a parent of young children. You love spending time with your family, and you have the patience and energy to cook healthy meals from scratch every day and to arrange spontaneous adventures and play dates at weekends. After brain injury, you're shouting at the kids all the time, can't stand the constant noise, and need to plan for a week before a trip to the playground.

What might you begin to conclude about yourself? How will you think about your future? How confident will you feel to try new things, or consider new, unfamiliar ways of doing things? How will these experiences be integrated into your self-system? Will these experiences activate identities from your store of experiences that depict you in a positive or negative light? Will you experience your behaviors and reactions as in keeping with your notion of yourself or at odds with that? All of these questions need to be kept in mind during rehabilitation.

As well as encountering cognitive, physical, and emotional changes, many people experience changes to motivation after brain injury—whether as a result of organic damage to drive systems, or of mood changes or executive dysfunction (Tyerman & King, 2009). Understanding the factors that influence a person's motivation, and how these may change after brain injury, can also support work on identity change. Kielhofner (2008) suggests that motivation is influenced by a person's core values, interests, and sense of capacity. A range of questions can be used to explore clients' motivation both before and after their injury; some things may have changed, but they may also find some constants. Which key roles, values, and interests motivate them, then and now? How has their injury affected their ability to live and express these values each day? What are their usual habits and patterns of occupation? What are their strengths and challenges from both physical and cognitive perspectives?

It is important to note that family members, friends, and spouses/partners of clients can also experience significant identity change as they become drawn into taking on the caregiver role. This role may be experienced as consistent with some aspects of identity, but at odds with their identity in their relationships with the clients. This discrepancy can underlie significant challenges with many aspects of life, including practical day-to-day arrangements, finance, child care, and sex/intimacy.

REHABILITATION: THE EVIDENCE

There is a growing evidence base for the importance of integrating identity work into brain injury rehabilitation, and for the potential effects of different rehabilitation approaches on self-concept, although findings are mixed and the methodological quality of studies to date has not always been very strong (Ownsworth & Haslam, 2014). Ownsworth and Haslam's (2014) review suggests that activity-based rehabilitation, cognitive rehabilitation, family support approaches, and psychotherapeutic approaches may all bring about changes in self-concept. However, this was not the case for all the studies they reviewed. There has been one good-quality trial of holistic or comprehensive neuropsychological rehabilitation (Cicerone et al., 2011) that was explicitly concerned with addressing identity change. Although this trial provided evidence of good outcomes across a range of measures, outcomes in terms of identity change were not measured.

MODELS OF IDENTITY

The "Y-shaped model" (Gracey, Evans, & Malley, 2009) suggests that we can best understand someone's struggles after brain injury (whether these struggles are characterized as depression, anger, or lack of insight) in terms of a "threat to self"—an underlying negative experience associated with experiencing oneself as fundamentally different from how one "should" be (see Figure 9.1). Often this experience is described in terms of discrepancy between the "old" or "ideal" self and the "current" self. People describe a sense of loss of self; a sense of being (in one client's words) "a was," not "an am" (Dewar & Gracey, 2007); or a feeling of disconnection as their acquired impairments affect their functional activity and relationships. The diagram of the model provided in Handout 9.1 can be used as a concrete introduction to discussing identity discrepancy with a client.

Ownsworth's (2014) model provides an account that also links changes in everyday life after brain injury to possible self-discrepancy and sense of threat to self. Particularly in the context of poor coping skills or low self-efficacy, this linkage could lead to further ultimately unhelpful consequences in day-to-day life, such as loss of friendships or withdrawal from activities.

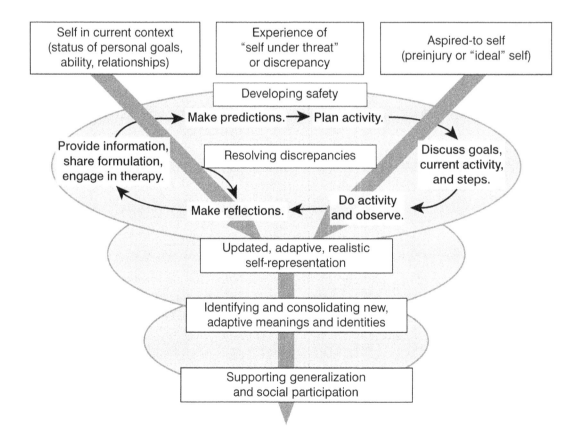

FIGURE 9.1. The full version of the Y-shaped model. Adapted by permission of Cambridge University Press from Wilson, Gracey, Malley, Bateman, and Evans (2009).

The "life thread model" (Ellis-Hill, Payne, & Ward, 2008) provides a similar account, suggesting that our lives are made up of multiple "narrative strands" like the strands in a piece of rope. Acquired brain injury (ABI) can cut some of these threads, and people may experience a sense of loss or disconnection that can influence well-being and confidence.

EXPLORING IDENTITY AND ITS DISRUPTION WITH CLIENTS

Rehabilitation can aim to help persons with brain injury and those around them develop a sense of themselves as being valued and having meaningful lives in which their postinjury situations are integrated into their identities. Engaging in cycles of doing and reflecting can reduce the sense of discrepancy and help to rebuild a "new me" after injury; it can address postinjury changes while at the same time supporting connection with enduring aspects of identity, such as values and beliefs.

There are three stages to working with identity in rehabilitation:

1. Understanding the past: Getting to know a person in the context of the person's life story.
2. Understanding the present: Evaluating the postinjury "landscape."
3. Mapping the future: Supporting the person's reengagement in meaningful activity, as a route to investing in a desired future self.

These stages and the examples of activities described below should ideally be carried out alongside other rehabilitation activities. For example, before current goals are discussed, it may help to reflect on the person's life to date. Plans for achieving goals should take the person's emotional and motivational landscape into account.

Understanding the Person in the Context of His or Her Life Story

The first thing we need to do as rehabilitation professionals is to understand each individual's life prior to and following the brain injury. We all live in worlds shaped by our past experiences, personal values, hopes, and fears. We need to develop an understanding of not only the reality of clients' lives (including relationships, resources, activities, and constraints), but also their perceptions of this reality (such as their sense of discrepancy vs. connectedness or confusion vs. coherence), so that we can better understand the threats to self the clients are experiencing.

Timelines

Drawing a series of timelines, each representing a different aspect of a person's life (e.g., school, work, family, friends), can provide a structured way for the person to explain his or her preinjury life. You could go on to consider which threads have continued after the injury, and which may have been broken or damaged, in the context of assessing current challenges and identifying goals. A timeline need not be limited to a simple linear measure: One client with a passion for horses created a three-dimensional show-jumping course to summarize the stages of her life; another chose to create a snake, with key images and words from his past in different sections of the animal's body; a third built a large wooden cube, with each surface representing a key life phase. The narrative "tree of life" approach can also provide a more dynamic, less linear way of developing a timeline. Encouraging each client to create a timeline in a personally meaningful way is the key here.

It is important to maintain a sense of curiosity and respect for the unknown during this work, and thus to try to make open-ended requests wherever possible—for instance, "Tell me about your life before your accident," "Describe three key events in your life," or "If your life was a play, what would be the key events, and who would be the main characters?" Clients with memory problems may benefit from using photographs or objects from their lives to recall past events; working with family members to collect supporting material can be invaluable here. Whatever approach you choose to take, encourage the clients to focus on their felt experiences of the events, rather than simply on what happened.

Understanding the Postinjury Landscape

Timeline work can help you to understand each client's back story, which inevitably has a major impact on the "landscape" in which the client lives at present. Changes brought by brain injury can significantly alter this landscape: Reduced physical and cognitive abilities and changing emotional reactions can act as barriers to meaningful participation, just as road construction, detours, and heavy traffic can disrupt a road trip. The activities throughout this workbook help clients to explore these areas of challenge.

Exploring Emotion

Handout 9.2 can be used to help clients and their families explore how their understandable emotional reactions to the threats to self resulting from brain injury can end up creating even more difficulties in the longer term—leading to what we call a vicious daisy of unhelpful threat-maintaining cycles. This handout may be particularly helpful for clients who indicate some ambivalence about making the changes needed to move forward with goals. It is important to try to understand emotional and behavioral consequences as arising from activation of the brain's threat system, and to try to develop a working relationship that focuses on (at least) one of the person's preinjury identities. This can help to foster safety, understanding, and a sense of familiarity and continuity. It may be necessary to collect information about specific "hot" situations or triggers, or to help a client use behavioral experiments as active tests of negative predictions in certain situations (for more guidance on behavioral experiments, see Winegardner, Chapter 5, and Ford, Chapter 8, this volume). There may also be supportive factors that can make the journey smoother, such as acceptance by key people in clients' lives, or moment-to-moment experiences of competence experienced with the use of compensatory strategies. Understanding both the barriers and supports in the postinjury landscape will support clients in moving forward with life and rebuilding identity after brain injury.

Exploring Motivation

Developing an understanding of a client's motivation after brain injury can be supported by a range of assessment questionnaires based on the "Model of Human Occupation" (Kielhofner, 2008), which are available online (*www.cade.uic.edu/moho*). The Modified Interest Checklist, Roles Questionnaire, and Occupational Questionnaire are available free of charge, whereas the Volitional Questionnaire and the Occupational Performance History Interview 2 can be purchased.

You can use the card-sorting activity provided in Handout 9.3 with clients to explore the values that are important to them in life. Ask them to sort the cards into categories according to whether they are very important or very unimportant to them. Then have them consider what kinds of activities or occupations in their current daily routines allow them to express these values.

Handout 9.4 can serve as a starting point for discussing changing roles within the family unit. It is best to have a client and family members complete this handout together, and to be prepared for some negotiation.

Use Handout 9.5 to help clients explore their motivation for engaging in certain occupations. Ask them to choose one activity they enjoy, and one they do not enjoy, and to consider these questions:

- Environment: Where do I do it, and with whom? Do I use any tools/equipment?
- Habituation: When/how often do I do it?
- Values: How obligated do I feel to do this? How important is it? Do I meet my own standards for the task?
- Personal causation: How confident am I in my abilities? How confident am I that I will succeed?
- Outcomes, thoughts, and feelings: What do I like/dislike about it? Do I enjoy it? How satisfying is it?

According to Kielhofner (2008, p. 37), "a negative sense of capacity can be even more disabling than the impairments on which it is based." Therefore, it is crucial that we understand clients' perceptions of their own abilities. Working either with individual clients or groups, make three different activities available (one suggestion might be playing a simple mobile phone game, drawing a picture, or playing pool or table tennis). You will need to tailor the activities to your clients' abilities, but ensure that each client is offered a variety of task types. Then, using Handout 9.6, ask clients to provide predicted and actual ratings for their ability, confidence, and enjoyment when completing each activity.

Identity Mapping

Mark Ylvisaker (2008) has proposed "identity mapping" as a practical exercise that can help to start the process of understanding clients and their present situation. Identity mapping is based on the belief that we all make meaning out of the materials available to us. However, we each have a different sense of meaning; what may be meaningful to one person may seem meaningless to another. Ylvisaker has suggested that identity is therefore defined by the personally meaningful activities an individual participates in, along with values, cultural beliefs, and other characteristics. Through pursuing personally meaningful goals, the individual creates constructive meaning. Rehabilitation professionals are therefore active collaborators in the process of constructing a compelling and satisfying sense of self.

Identity maps may be constructed at different time points in rehabilitation, depending on the purpose of the activity.

* *Mapping the discrepancy.* Mapping the perceived discrepancy in detail is useful at the start of rehabilitation, as it can allow each individual to reflect on this throughout and therefore to recognize when the discrepancy is decreasing. A pair of diagrams resembling spider webs, in which clients describe themselves before and after the injury, can be a simple way to make the felt discrepancy visible.

* *Carving out a new identity.* Some individuals may find it difficult to develop a sense of what their identity may look like in the future. This may go along with difficulty in finding goals for rehabilitation. As noted earlier in the chapter, this process can be particularly challenging for clients who suffered their injury at younger ages, when they were in the process of forming their adult identities. In this scenario, identity maps can be a useful way of supporting goal setting. For example, Figure 9.2 shows an identity map entitled "The man I want to be." The client chose to use graffiti, which was a particular art form he enjoyed. He was able to produce the diagram despite having difficulty identifying the goals he wanted to focus on in rehabilitation.

* *Developing roles.* Identity maps can also support clients in organizing and understanding the relationships between different roles they fulfill as part of their identities. In the example shown in Figure 9.3, the client's vocational rehabilitation goal involved exploring a new profession (personal trainer). Over time, an additional perceived identity—that of a worker/professional—became part of his sense of self.

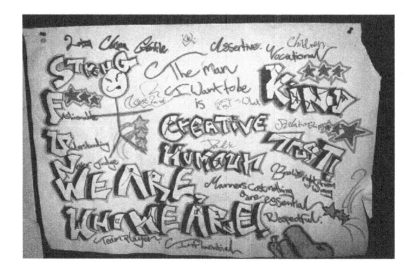

FIGURE 9.2. "The man I want to be": Developing an identity map by using graffiti.

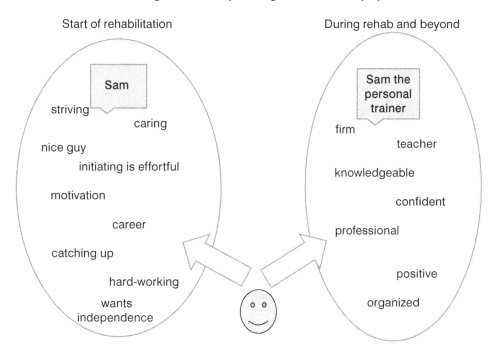

FIGURE 9.3. "Sam the personal trainer": Exploring a new identity in vocational rehabilitation.

• *Metaphor.* Ylvisaker (2008) suggests that identity mapping may also include a component in which a client describes his or her identity through a metaphor (e.g., a client wishing to be a mother/homemaker may think of herself as "Susan as a domestic goddess"). The metaphor may be someone the client identifies with or aspires to emulate (i.e., a hero or heroine) and can therefore be someone the client knows personally, a fictitious character, or a celebrity or public figure. It can also be someone who embodies characteristics the client does *not* aspire to. An example of the latter type of metaphor is given in Figure 9.4. Tommy Cooper was a comedian popular in Britain in the 1970s, and drawing an identity map of himself as Tommy Cooper enabled clear identification of goals for this client.

• *Identifying goals.* As the preceding example suggests, adding the metaphor component can help a client to identify goals to develop, as well as positive personal characteristics. Another example is of a client who used a different name when socializing with his friends at the pub. Through identity mapping, he was able to explore the ways in which this alter ego served as an important part of his coping strategy—and to set the goal of developing his coping skills further.

Engaging in Activities That Connect with Underlying Values and Meanings

To a great extent, we human beings define ourselves by what we do. Whether we are chatting to old friends, meeting new people at a party, or using social media, our conversations often focus on what we do for a living, what we enjoy doing in our spare time, or what we

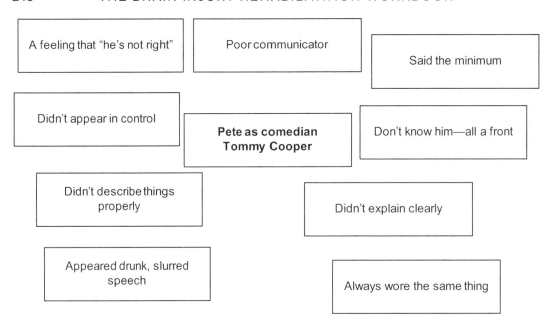

FIGURE 9.4. "Becoming Tommy Cooper": Using metaphor to explore identity reconstruction.

have been up to recently. This anecdotal observation is supported by literature from occupational science and occupational therapy, and is in keeping with Conway's (2005) memory self-system model described earlier. Christiansen (1999) views occupation as a "principal means through which people develop and express their personal identities." Kielhofner (2008) observes that "When people work, play and perform [activities of daily living], they shape their capacities, patterns of acting, self-perceptions and comprehension of our world . . . people author their own development through what they do." When an individual's occupational participation is affected by illness or injury, it is inevitable that the person's identity is affected. For some, loss of a particularly meaningful role or activity can feel like a total loss of identity, as in the case of a young man who has had a traumatic brain injury (TBI) and can no longer drive. One of the aims of brain injury rehabilitation is to support occupational adaptation—or, as Kielhofner describes it, "the construction of a positive occupational identity, achieving occupational competence over time in the context of one's environment." To look at this another way, by connecting with what an activity means to a person, rehabilitation can support people with ABI in finding other things to do to express their core values, and thus to fill the void that can be left after injury. This is represented in the "do" and "reflect" stages of the Y-shaped model.

Occupational Experiments

Engaging in and reflecting on occupational experiences—with consideration of all the factors affecting occupational performance—can act as a vehicle for changing occupational identity (Kielhofner, 2008). Handout 9.7 offers an occupational experiment tool, which has been adapted from a standard behavioral experiment sheet; Handout 9.8 provides questions to guide reflection on such an experiment from an occupation-focused perspective (Martin-Saez, Winson, Malley, Brentnall, & Runcie, 2012). Some clients may require support to consider an objective view of what actually happened, as well as their felt experience; accordingly, these two handouts are written to be used by a client and clinician working together.

Goal Ladders

Clients may require a graded approach to selecting appropriate activities to explore. Some activities may be too threatening at a given point in time. The "comfort zones" exercise provided in Handout 9.9 can be used to plot which activities feel most and least accessible. For example, a client who wrote poetry had a dream of performing at an open-mic night. When the comfort zones exercise was completed at the start of her therapy program, this dream felt impossible to her. Reading a poem to the therapist felt less threatening, and performing her work in front of her rehabilitation group lay somewhere in between. As she progressed, this exercise was revisited from time to time; the process helped her to notice that her feelings were changing as she developed confidence. She eventually achieved her goal of performing her poetry in public.

Projects

Ylvisaker (2003) has proposed that projects can be positive vehicles for assisting identity reconstruction. Projects based on personally meaningful goals and directed toward concrete outcomes can offer opportunities to implement and consolidate strategies and entrench a positive identity. An ideal project encourages a felt sense of contributing to others through both the content and process involved. The content of the project offers opportunities for acquiring new learning or drawing on preinjury knowledge. Simultaneously, the process of starting a project and working on it over a period of time offers opportunities for repetitive practice of various cognitive skills (memory, planning, time management, organization, initiation, problem solving, and goal management), and thereby for consolidation of these skills in a real-life context. Successful projects have a positive impact on self-esteem and confidence, which may facilitate motivation, and these effects may generalize into other areas of the individual's life. Examples of projects clients have undertaken are described below.

- Goal: To develop skills to support the achievement of a desired role as a fitness instructor.
- Plans:
  - Conduct a fitness assessment interview.
  - Instruct individual fitness programs.
  - Run a fitness class with volunteers.
  - Meet weekly with a mentor (a professional personal trainer).

  The project involved developing a range of strategies to achieve these plans, thereby tapping into the areas of communication (interviewing, giving instructions effectively), cognition (initiation, planning/time management), and mood. Video feedback and

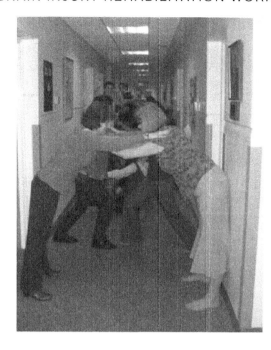

FIGURE 9.5. Exercise classes for the rehabilitation team: Realizing a client's desired role as a personal trainer through action.

behavior rating scales supported the client's development over time. The project helped the client to integrate the new role (personal trainer) into his original identity. Practical activities (see Figure 9.5 for an example) allowed him to have the experience of "feeling" like a personal trainer, which made the whole project more meaningful.

Project work can also be carried out in groups; this can be particularly useful for clients hoping to return to work. In a group of three, each person was given the opportunity to lead a particular project over a 3-month period.

- Goal: To develop project leadership skills with the aim of returning to work.
- Plans:
  - Plan a Christmas party.
  - Produce a newsletter.
  - Organize a fund-raising event.

Each project ran over a 4-week period, with a different person acting as project leader each time. The clients needed to use a variety of communication strategies to facilitate working in a team, managing disagreements, and giving feedback in order to achieve the desired outcome for each project. The cognitive and executive functioning strategies required included planning, Stop/Think, the Goal Management Framework (GMF), and Time Pressure Management (TPM) (see Winegardner, Chapter 5). These scenarios raised many challenges, but allowed patterns of behavior to be identified and difficulties to be addressed before these clients entered a real-life return-to-work situation.

- Goal: To explore new meaningful activities.
- Plans:
  - Attend a jewelry-making class in a "safe" group.
  - Plan a jewelry sale in the hospital.
  - Arrange a jewelry sale at home for friends and family members.

As a result of her brain injury, this client was unable to return to her role as a nurse in the health sector. However, she longed to find a meaningful activity that she could do in her own home, which could also generate income. She was very interested in jewelry making, but lacked confidence that she would be able to learn this skill, much less earn money from it. The project started with a shared, safe learning environment: Together, staff members and the client attended a jewelry-making course. This safety allowed her to excel at the skill and encouraged her to take her learning further. The next step— arranging a jewelry sale within the hospital (see Figure 9.6)—provided the client and her team with a vehicle for implementing planning and organizing strategies in a supported way, which allowed the stall to succeed. Although not everything went according to plan, following through on the plans enabled the client to learn even when some things went wrong. This learning was much more powerful in the context of a project that was personally meaningful to the client. The process supported her to develop a positive identity as someone who was capable of achieving, despite not being able to fulfill the same role as before her injury.

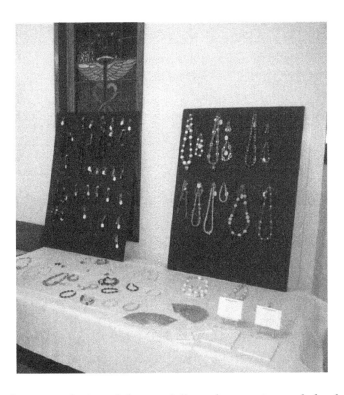

FIGURE 9.6. Making it real: Consolidating skills and strategies, and developing confidence, through a meaningful project (a jewelry sale in the hospital).

- Goal: To explore meaningful vocational opportunities.
- Plans:
  - Explore values relating to work.
  - Run an art class.
  - Produce pet portraits.

A client working in an administrative job was struggling to return to work after a subarachnoid hemorrhage. She was unable to perform tasks to the required standard and was frequently in conflict with her colleagues, with negative consequences for her self-esteem: "I'm no good at anything, and I don't feel 'heard.'" Assessment revealed that although many of the client's cognitive skills were good, she had difficulty with motivation and responsibility, along with a weak pattern of occupation and inaccurate appraisal of her own skills. In addition, neither the role nor the working environment allowed her to express her core values of fairness, freedom, and creativity, and she clearly identified her frustration with this in her individual therapy sessions.

The intervention focused on exploring working environments that might be a better fit for the client's needs. She was an enthusiastic artist, so the first project involved running a drawing class for staff and clients. After an initial session that was rather lacking in structure and guidance from the "teacher," feedback from the "students" helped identify the need for a lesson plan and an approach that focused on supporting others as opposed to simply enjoying drawing herself. Seeing her students' confidence develop under her guidance brought a sense of satisfaction, with the result that the client began to take increased responsibility for the sessions by the end of the intervention. A further project involved exploring the possibility of drawing pet portraits; the client was supported to interview potential "customers" to gain a sense of their needs and their pets' personalities, and then to use scheduling and self-management techniques to produce portraits by certain deadlines.

Learning from these projects gave the client the confidence to resign from her existing job, and to target her subsequent job search to areas more congruent with her current values and abilities.

Self-Coaching and Mentoring

Ylvisaker (2008) has also referred to "self-coaching" as a useful tool for guiding behavior. Self-talk in this context has a regulatory function and can be triggered by personally relevant environmental events or contexts. The general goal of self-talk is to improve behavior by decreasing impulsive and reactive behavior. The encouraged control over behavior can facilitate a positive sense of self, and takes place alongside social and vocational participation.

The coaching idea can be extended to include others. An identified mentor can support a client through a particular project or activities. Mentors can be identified according to the expertise they bring, and may therefore include volunteers or individuals identified in vocational or voluntary placements.

ADDRESSING COGNITIVE AND OTHER BARRIERS

The focus of the preceding chapters of this book is on helping clients to develop a shared understanding of their relative strengths and challenges, and to explore strategies to overcome their difficulties. Some cognitive impairments may make it harder for clients to update their identities. Diaries, social scaffolding, and the use of technology such as wearable "life-logging" cameras (such as Autographer or Narrative Clip) can help clients to monitor the changes in themselves, and to share with others. Clients can use Handout 9.10 to record what they learn about themselves during therapy.

As the projects described above demonstrate, it is most effective to carry out identity work in meaningful contexts—ones that enable clients to explore how they can continue to live out their most cherished roles and values after brain injury. A clear, shared understanding of abilities means that activities can be adapted to accommodate individual differences and even to exploit strengths in a compensatory approach. For example, for someone with significant prospective memory difficulties in the context of good semantic memory, setting up a meaningful project that creates lots of opportunities to practice prospective memory strategies whilst allowing the client to demonstrate semantic knowledge (perhaps through writing an article or newsletter) can build confidence while simultaneously developing coping skills.

It is not enough to draw on projects, goal ladders, and experiments to facilitate identity reconstruction. These tools also need to be personalized to individual clients' interests, strengths, and challenges, in order for their experience to be meaningful *and* enriching.

REFERENCES

Christiansen, C. (1999). Defining lives: Occupation as identity. An essay on competence, coherence, and the creation of meaning. *American Journal of Occupational Therapy, 53,* 547–558.

Cicerone, K. D., Langenbahn, D. M., Braden, C., Malec, J. F., Kalmar, K., Fraas, M., . . . Ashman, T. (2011). Evidence-based cognitive rehabilitation: Updated review of the literature from 2003 through 2008. *Archives of Physical Medicine and Rehabilitation, 92*(4), 519–530.

Conway, M. (2005). Memory and the self. *Journal of Memory and Language, 53*(4), 594–628.

Damasio, A. (2000). *The feeling of what happens: Body and emotion in the making of consciousness.* New York: Mariner Books.

Damasio, A. (2005). *Descartes' error: Emotion, reason, and the human brain.* New York: Penguin.

Dewar, B.-K., & Gracey, F. (2007). 'Am not was': Cognitive-behavioural therapy for adjustment and identity change following herpes simplex encephalitis. *Neuropsychological Rehabilitation, 17*(4–5), 602–620.

Ellis-Hill, C., Payne, S., & Ward, C. (2008). Using stroke to explore the life thread model: An alternative approach to understanding rehabilitation following an acquired disability. *Disability and Rehabilitation, 30*(2), 150–159.

Gracey, F., Evans, J. J., & Malley, D. (2009). Capturing process and outcome in complex rehabilitation interventions: A 'Y-shaped' model. *Neuropsychological Rehabilitation, 19*(6), 867–890.

Gracey, F., Longworth, C. E., & Psaila, K. (2015). A provisional transdiagnostic cognitive behavioural model of post brain injury emotional adjustment. *Neuro-Disability and Psychotherapy, 3*(2), 154–185.

Kielhofner, G. (2008). *Model of human occupation: Theory and application.* Baltimore: Lippincott Williams & Wilkins.

LeDoux, J. (1998). *The emotional brain: The mysterious underpinnings of emotional life.* New York: Simon & Schuster.

Martin-Saez, M., Winson, R. W. H., Malley, D., Brentnall, S., & Runcie, R. (2012). *Reconstructing identity through occupational participation.* Poster presented at the International Brain Injury Association 9th World Congress, Edinburgh, UK.

Ownsworth, T. (2014). *Self-identity after brain injury.* Hove, UK: Psychology Press.

Ownsworth, T., & Haslam, C. (2014). Impact of rehabilitation on self-concept following traumatic brain injury: An exploratory systematic review of intervention methodology and efficacy. *Neuropsychological Rehabilitation, 26*(1), 1–35.

Tyerman, A., & King, N. S. (Eds.). (2009). *Psychological approaches to rehabilitation after traumatic brain injury.* Oxford, UK: Blackwell.

Wilson, B. A., Gracey, F., Malley, D., Bateman, A., & Evans, J. J. (2009). The Oliver Zangwill Centre approach to neuropsychological rehabilitation. In B. A. Wilson, F. Gracey, J. J. Evans, & A. Bateman, *Neuropsychological rehabilitation: Theory, models, therapy and outcome.* Cambridge, UK: Cambridge University Press.

Yeates, G. N., Gracey, F., & McGrath, J. C. (2008). A biopsychosocial deconstruction of 'personality change' following acquired brain injury. *Neuropsychological Rehabilitation, 18*(5–6), 566–589.

Ylvisaker, M. (2003). Context-sensitive cognitive rehabilitation after brain injury: Theory and practice. *Brain Impairment, 4*(1), 1–16.

Ylvisaker, M. (2008). Metaphoric identity mapping: Facilitating goal setting and engagement in rehabilitation after traumatic brain injury. *Neuropsychological Rehabilitation, 18*(5–6), 713–741.

Ylvisaker, M., & Feeney, T. (2000). Reconstruction of identity after brain injury. *Brain Impairment, 1*(1), 2–28.

FURTHER READING

Jetten, J., Haslam, C., & Haslam, S. A. (Eds.). (2012). *The social cure: Identity, health and well-being.* Hove, UK: Psychology Press.

The Y-Shaped Model of Identity Change in Rehabilitation

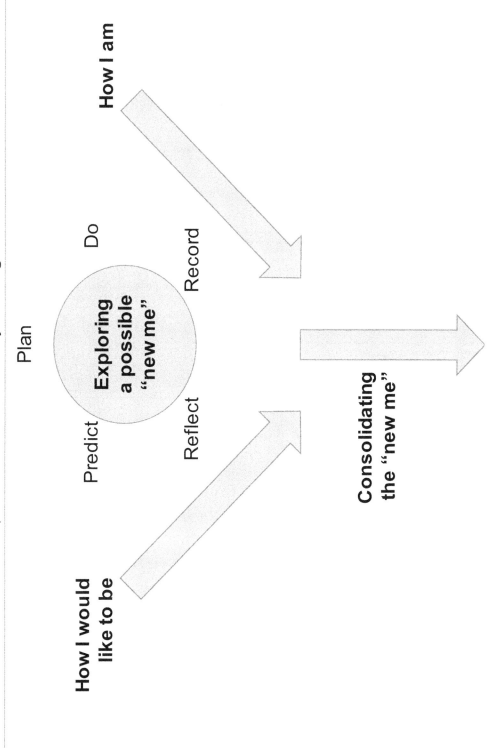

Plan

Do

Predict

Record

Reflect

Exploring a possible "new me"

How I am

How I would like to be

Consolidating the "new me"

Adapted by permission of Cambridge University Press from Wilson, Gracey, Malley, Bateman, and Evans (2009).

From *The Brain Injury Rehabilitation Workbook*, edited by Rachel Winson, Barbara A. Wilson, and Andrew Bateman. Copyright © 2017 The Guilford Press. Permission to photocopy this handout is granted to purchasers of this book for personal use or for use with individual clients (see copyright page for details). Purchasers can download additional copies of this handout (see the box at the end of the table of contents).

The "Vicious Daisy" Cycle

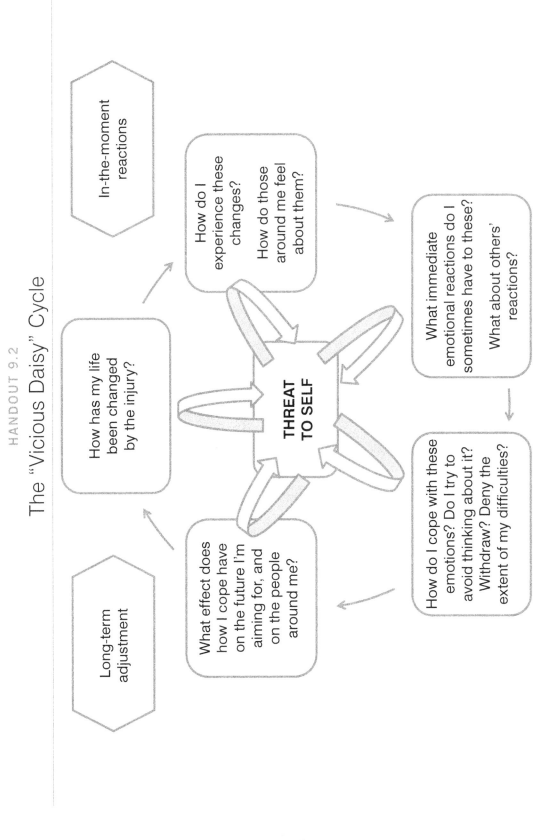

In-the-moment reactions

How do I experience these changes?

How do those around me feel about them?

What immediate emotional reactions do I sometimes have to these?

What about others' reactions?

How has my life been changed by the injury?

THREAT TO SELF

How do I cope with these emotions? Do I try to avoid thinking about it? Withdraw? Deny the extent of my difficulties?

Long-term adjustment

What effect does how I cope have on the future I'm aiming for, and on the people around me?

From Gracey, Longworth, and Psaila (2015). Reprinted with kind permission of Karnac books.

Personal Values

Cut along the dotted lines to create a card for each word. Then sort the cards according to whether the words are important or not important to you.

acceptance	accuracy	achievement	adventure	attractiveness
authority	autonomy	beauty	caring	challenge
change	comfort	commitment	compassion	contribution
cooperation	courtesy	creativity	dependability	duty
ecology	excitement	faithfulness	fame	family
fitness	flexibility	forgiveness	friendship	fun
generosity	genuineness	God's will	growth	health
helpfulness	honesty	hope	humility	humor
independence	inner peace	industry	intimacy	justice
knowledge	leisure	love	mastery	mindfulness
moderation	monogamy	nonconformity	nurturing	openness
order	passion	pleasure	popularity	power
purpose	rationality	realism	responsibility	risk
romance	safety	self-acceptance	self-control	self-esteem
self-knowledge	sexuality	simplicity	solitude	spirituality
stability	tolerance	tradition	virtue	wealth
world peace				

Adapted from W. R. Miller, J. C'de Baca, D. B. Matthews, and P. L. Wilbourne, University of New Mexico (2001). In the public domain.

From *The Brain Injury Rehabilitation Workbook*, edited by Rachel Winson, Barbara A. Wilson, and Andrew Bateman. Copyright © 2017 The Guilford Press. Permission to photocopy this handout is granted to purchasers of this book for personal use or for use with individual clients (see copyright page for details). Purchasers can download additional copies of this handout (see the box at the end of the table of contents).

Family Roles

Who completed these tasks in the past (before the brain injury)? Who does them now? Who will do them in the future?

Activity	Past	Now	Future
Looking after children			
Planning things to do as a family			
Preparing lunch			
Preparing evening meals			
Cleaning			
Laundry			
Home repairs			
Budgeting			
Making appointments			
Shopping (big stores)			
Shopping (smaller stores)			
Handling correspondence			
Car maintenance			
Paying bills			
Gardening/yard work			
Taking out trash and recycling			
Looking after pets			

From *The Brain Injury Rehabilitation Workbook*, edited by Rachel Winson, Barbara A. Wilson, and Andrew Bateman. Copyright © 2017 The Guilford Press. Permission to photocopy this handout is granted to purchasers of this book for personal use or for use with individual clients (see copyright page for details). Purchasers can download additional copies of this handout (see the box at the end of the table of contents).

My Motivation: Why Do I Do What I Do?

How important is it to me?	
How confident am I in my abilities?	Who do I do it with?
What do I like/dislike about it?	When/how often do I do it?
How satisfying is it? (0–10)	

Activity

How confident am I that I will succeed and/or enjoy it? (0–10)

Do I enjoy it? (0–10)

Where do I do it?

Do I use any equipment?

To what extent do I feel I *should* do it?

Am I able to meet my own standards? (0–10)

Developed in collaboration with Maria Martin-Saez.

From *The Brain Injury Rehabilitation Workbook*, edited by Rachel Winson, Barbara A. Wilson, and Andrew Bateman. Copyright © 2017 The Guilford Press. Permission to photocopy this handout is granted to purchasers of this book for personal use or for use with individual clients (see copyright page for details). Purchasers can download additional copies of this handout (see the box at the end of the table of contents).

Predictions

On a scale of 1–10 (1 = terrible, 5 = not bad, 10 = excellent), please rate how well you think you will do on each activity (ability), how confident you think you will be while doing the activity (confidence), and how much you think you will enjoy it (enjoyment). These are your predicted ratings. Then, after you do each activity, use the same rating scale to rate your actual ability, confidence, and enjoyment.

Activity 1:

	Ability	Confidence	Enjoyment
Predicted			
Actual			

Activity 2:

	Ability	Confidence	Enjoyment
Predicted			
Actual			

Activity 3:

	Ability	Confidence	Enjoyment
Predicted			
Actual			

Developed in collaboration with Maria Martin-Saez.

From *The Brain Injury Rehabilitation Workbook*, edited by Rachel Winson, Barbara A. Wilson, and Andrew Bateman. Copyright © 2017 The Guilford Press. Permission to photocopy this handout is granted to purchasers of this book for personal use or for use with individual clients (see copyright page for details). Purchasers can download additional copies of this handout (see the box at the end of the table of contents).

Occupational Experiment

Description of activity	Feelings and thoughts before the activity	What actually happened— from both your and other people's viewpoints?	Your interpretation of the experience

Developed in collaboration with Maria Martin-Saez.

From *The Brain Injury Rehabilitation Workbook*, edited by Rachel Winson, Barbara A. Wilson, and Andrew Bateman. Copyright © 2017 The Guilford Press. Permission to photocopy this handout is granted to purchasers of this book for personal use or for use with individual clients (see copyright page for details). Purchasers can download additional copies of this handout (see the box at the end of the table of contents).

Questions and Observations for an Occupational Experiment

Questions	Observations
Volition (personal causation): Do you feel you have the abilities for doing this task? Do you feel your efforts will result in achieving your goal?	
Volition (values): Is this task important to you?	
Volition (interests): Will you enjoy doing this activity? Why or why not?	
Habituation (routines): What impact will the completion of this activity have on your daily routines?	
Habituation (roles): Do you feel this task is/could be your responsibility as part of your role as a____?	
Environment: What aspects of the environment (objects, people, space) will facilitate or restrict your performance?	

Developed in collaboration with Maria Martin-Saez.

From *The Brain Injury Rehabilitation Workbook*, edited by Rachel Winson, Barbara A. Wilson, and Andrew Bateman. Copyright © 2017 The Guilford Press. Permission to photocopy this handout is granted to purchasers of this book for personal use or for use with individual clients (see copyright page for details). Purchasers can download additional copies of this handout (see the box at the end of the table of contents).

Comfort Zones

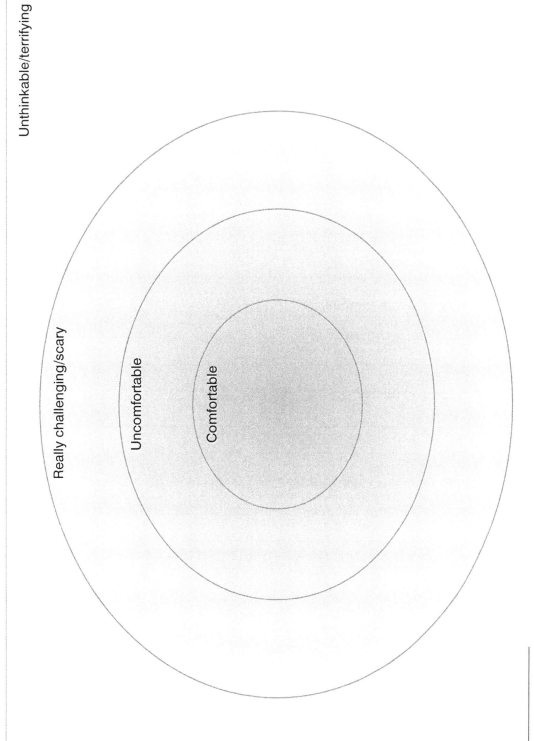

Unthinkable/terrifying

Really challenging/scary

Uncomfortable

Comfortable

From *The Brain Injury Rehabilitation Workbook*, edited by Rachel Winson, Barbara A. Wilson, and Andrew Bateman. Copyright © 2017 The Guilford Press. Permission to photocopy this handout is granted to purchasers of this book for personal use or for use with individual clients (see copyright page for details). Purchasers can download additional copies of this handout (see the box at the end of the table of contents).

How Do I See Myself?

We all have plans and aspirations about ourselves and what and where we want to be in our lives. A brain injury can result in many interruptions to plans and aspirations (such as changes in relationships, work, leisure, or socializing).

You might end up thinking about how you were before your injury and compare it to how you are now, asking yourself, "Why can't it be like it was? Why can't it be like I think it should be?" Responding to the items below may help you to think about your life before and after the brain injury, and to take stock of the strengths you still have, your values, and your sources of support.

Before my injury, I saw myself as: _____

_____

_____

Brain injury affected my life and my plans for the future in these ways: _____

_____

_____

Since my brain injury, I have seen myself as: _____

_____

_____

What are my strengths and values? _____

_____

_____

How do my strengths and values help to support the areas I have difficulties with? _____

_____

_____

These are the things and people that support my wellness: _____

_____

_____

These are the things and people that inspire me and remind me of my values: _____

_____

_____

From *The Brain Injury Rehabilitation Workbook*, edited by Rachel Winson, Barbara A. Wilson, and Andrew Bateman. Copyright © 2017 The Guilford Press. Permission to photocopy this handout is granted to purchasers of this book for personal use or for use with individual clients (see copyright page for details). Purchasers can download additional copies of this handout (see the box at the end of the table of contents).

CHAPTER 10

Working with Families after Brain Injury

Leyla Prince

BACKGROUND

Why should brain injury rehabilitation professionals be working with families? A client's father once described the impact of the brain injury on the family as "collateral damage." This is a military term, used for unintentional damage inflicted on bystanders near an intended target. The collateral damage in any situation, although regrettable, is often brushed aside as an unfortunate co-occurrence and seldom receives the attention it deserves. This father's use of the term was a vivid description of the position that many family members find themselves in when a loved one has suffered an acquired brain injury (ABI).

It is widely recognized that brain injury has a profound impact not only on the injured individual, but also on family and friends. The impact of brain injury on the family has been well documented over the past few decades (Brooks, 1991; Hall et al., 1994; Langlois, Rutland-Brown, & Wald, 2006), and it is widely accepted that the family shares the trauma and is a vital component of the rehabilitation process (Knight, Deveraux, & Godfrey, 1998; Oddy & Herbert, 2003; Bowen, 2007). Cognitive, emotional, physical, and communication impairments that arise after brain injury have an impact on what clients are able to do and how they think, feel, and communicate. These effects profoundly influence their ability to maintain roles and relationships (Bowen, Yeates, & Palmer, 2010).

As clinicians, we do have an important role to play in an individual's rehabilitation—but, as Lezak (1988) pointed out, brain injury is ultimately a family affair. After rehabilitation, clients go home to their families, and the family members are the ones who share the clients' experience of living with brain injury. Yeates (2009) clearly outlines the diverse and critical consequences for relatives of people with ABI, including low mood, caregiver strain/burden, and general psychological distress. Other common outcomes include significant challenges to psychological adjustment, sexual and relationship difficulties, and marital/couple strain and breakdown. Recent research has also shown that an increased sense of caregiver burden adversely affects the functioning of survivors after brain injury (Hsu, Kreutzer, & Menzel, 2009), and that encouraging families to engage in rehabilitation can maximize rehabilitation effectiveness (Lehan, Arango-Lasprilla, de los Reyes, & Quijano, 2012).

There is therefore abundant evidence that brain injury has a significant impact on both the individual and family. However, family intervention is not yet routinely integrated into neurorehabilitation in many settings. This chapter introduces some ideas—both old and new—that can underpin our approach to working with families, along with practical ideas that can be implemented in most settings to enhance the impact of neurorehabilitation. The practical ideas presented here by no means exhaust the possibilities, but ideally they will inspire clinicians to think more broadly when it comes to working with family members.

DEFINING "FAMILY"

> When everything goes to hell, the people who stand by you
> without flinching—they are your family.
> —BUTCHER (2006)

The meanings of the term "family" have changed significantly over the past few decades, with increasing variation even in the makeup of what was previously considered the nuclear family. Unmarried partners, single-sex partnerships, single-parent families, and nonrelatives as "family members" are now commonplace. There is also far greater diversity in people's expectations of different roles within a family.

As clinicians, we need to acknowledge that our ideas about who makes up a family are largely influenced by our own experiences of being part of a family and by the discourses inherent in our society at a given time (Dallos & Draper, 2010). It is important to acknowledge our own predispositions and then take the important step of finding out who makes up each individual's family. An individual's choice of "family members" may have less to do with who the person's blood relations are and more with who supports the person in everyday life. For example, a client who has lived independently of his or her parents for a significant time may be more likely to call on close friends for support. Although most people are likely to include their relatives in their immediate support network, it is important not to assume that this is always the case. The "family members" we work with should be identified by the client prior to any family assessment, and may include friends or significant others as well as blood relatives. This is even more important in situations where the persons with brain injury have cognitive or communication impairments that compromise their ability to articulate their views of "family." In addition to identifying who a client considers family members, it is essential to give consideration to meeting the needs of the client's children or other child relatives, as far as possible.

SYSTEMIC APPROACHES IN NEUROREHABILITATION

According to Oddy and Herbert (2003), there is a lack of theoretically guided and evidence-based family interventions for families of people with brain injury. Yeates (2009), however, has described a systemic family therapy approach to working with families in neuropsychological rehabilitation. As the term "systemic" indicates, adherents of this approach view the family as a system and acknowledge that external forces will have an impact on the system. Leber and Jenkins (1996) suggest that response patterns in the family system's previous functioning are activated when a traumatic event such as ABI occurs. It is important for the clinician and the family to develop a shared understanding of these responses during rehabilitation. Systemic approaches require approaching family work from a position of curiosity; it is important not to assume an understanding too quickly. However, families of individuals who have experienced brain injury often report that feeling understood is what they value most from clinicians. It is therefore important as a clinician to find a balance between helping a family to feel understood, and not attempting to be "the expert" on the family. A systemic approach involves facilitating conversations with a family that permit different perspectives to emerge, thereby allowing the family members to generate the solutions to their perceived problems.

Family life cycle theorists argue that families often experience difficulties when they are going through a transition or life cycle change, such as a member's leaving home, a birth, a death, or a divorce (Burnham, 1986). DePompei and Williams (1994) have suggested that when someone suffers a brain injury, this may lead to prolonged life cycle stages or even reversal of earlier changes. For example, a person with brain injury may need to move back home to live with parents after living independently or with a partner. Although this move may be driven by financial or practical reasons, parental roles are sometimes reclaimed and a partner may be excluded (DePompei & Williams, 1994). In other cases, although previously established patterns within a family may take hold during a crisis, these are not always helpful and can threaten stability. For example, a husband and wife who were separated were reunited through the need for care after one partner suffered a brain injury. In this case, a life cycle change (separation/divorce) was reversed, but not by repair of the relationship difficulties. It is therefore important to consider the stage of the family life cycle at the time of the ABI and how this may be affected by the injury.

Rolland (1999) has proposed a family systems–illness model in which the unfolding of a chronic disorder is viewed in a developmental context with three intertwining, evolving "threads": the life cycles of the illness, of the individual with the illness, and of the family. Rolland also proposes that different tasks and challenges face families at three different time phases in the development of illness; he describes these phases as "crisis," "chronic," and "terminal." Within brain injury (the illness thread, to use Rolland's term), the crisis phase involves acute onset; affective and practical changes occur in a short time period. Family members are placed under immense pressure in highly charged emotional situations, often exchange roles and solve problems flexibly, and use outside resources.

However, according to this model, the relapsing or episodic nature of the brain injury becomes apparent in the chronic phase. Family members are strained by the frequency of transitions between crisis and noncrisis, as well as by the uncertainty of the future of the brain injury—what degree of functioning will be recovered and what will be permanently lost. Brain injury can also bring a level of long-term disability (e.g., impairment of cognition). The extent of long-term disability will affect the degree of family stress. Rolland proposes that by considering the impact on the family at these different time phases of illness, and by considering the family's needs from the perspective of the three life cycles (those of the illness, the individual, and the family), we can better anticipate the family's needs at different stages after the injury.

The outcome of brain injury involves loss of identity and other losses that change the individual. These losses have been likened to the losses one may experience when someone has died. However, the fundamental difference is the continued physical presence of the person with the injury, which interferes with a family's attempts to adjust to the losses (Hall et al., 1994). If we think about this experience in terms of the family systems–illness framework, the family remains in the chronic phase, but the sense of loss can be experienced in every stage of illness in different ways.

The Y-shaped process model developed by Wilson, Gracey, Malley, Evans, and Bateman (2009) is based on the notion that there is a discrepancy between preinjury identity and postinjury reality, causing a catastrophic emotional reaction (Ben-Yishay, 2000) in response to the threat of postinjury changes. The model may be applied to the family in a similar way: There is a discrepancy between the preinjury family identity and the postinjury reality of the family system living with the brain injury. In rehabilitation, the aim is for clients to integrate the new reality of their postinjury lives with their preinjury representations of themselves, others, and the world. For the clients' families, this process is duplicated as they find a way of being in the future, in the context of the ABI and its consequences. More information on the Y-shaped model is provided by Gracey, Prince, and Winson in Chapter 9 of this book (see especially Handout 9.1).

In systemic terms, Johnson and McCown (1997) describe family members as poorly prepared to reincorporate the person with brain injury back into the family system, and suggest that the process of reintegration causes systemic disruptions that affect the person with brain injury and the family in a mutually causational pattern. Significantly, contemporary systemic family therapy also considers the contextual influences on the family, and includes the influence of clinicians and how they may shape or influence a family system. External contextual issues affect the family system, and, depending on the nature of the issue, can receive greater privilege than rehabilitation at any given time. It is important to be aware of these issues and to consider these as part of the "bigger picture." For example, an ongoing legal case, outside the control of the individual with brain injury or the family, can affect the individual's and family's sense of control of their lives (both financially and in terms of planning for the future). Similarly, changes in vocational status can bring about redistribution of roles, leading to sometimes unwanted identity change for both the individual and the family. These secondary consequences of brain injury have an enormous impact on the family system, and although such changes are often due to necessity and are acknowledged as such, they can be difficult to accept. It is therefore essential as clinicians to broaden our views in our bid to support our clients and their families.

FINDING OUT ABOUT THE FAMILY AND ITS MEMBERS' NEEDS

Before any specific family intervention is offered, it may be prudent to spend some time finding out about a client's family through a family assessment interview. This can be done with or without the client, depending on the circumstances. A family assessment interview has two aims—first, to find out who makes up the family of the person with brain injury; and, second, to explore any support needs that the family might have. In some cases, the client may not have family members involved in his or her support, and then it is important to be aware of who supports the client when the person is not having rehabilitation.

One way of finding out who is considered "family" is drawing a genogram with the client and the family members. Try to include three generations if possible, as well as close friends and people from the client's social and professional networks. The process of drawing a genogram or a family tree allows other information about the family practices and relationships to filter through. Simply having time to talk about the family can be immensely helpful; most of the conversations in rehabilitation are focused on the person with brain injury, so the family interview may be the first opportunity for others to express their views. This discussion can be a useful starting point for exploring any particular stress points for the family, which may indicate the kinds of support the family needs now and may need later. Such issues may be harder to identify in joint sessions focusing on the person with brain injury; the opportunity to discuss the experiences of the rest of the family is therefore most valuable.

Other useful ways of determining the needs of the family include the use of formal questionnaires. Kreutzer, Marwitz, Godwin, and Arango-Lasprilla (2010) have reported a list of commonly encountered family problems after ABI; it can be helpful to keep this list handy during an initial interview. The commonly experienced problems tend to center around difficulties in relation to understanding the injury and emotional difficulties relating to support needs. This exercise enables families to rate the importance of different problem areas, which can help the rehabilitation team to identify which areas will require intervention first. For example, if "feeling confused about the consequences of the injury" is rated highly, this suggests that starting with education about brain injury and its consequences would be appropriate. It may also be helpful to use the Dyadic Adjustment Scale (Spanier, 1976, 1989), a self-report measure of relationship adjustment. Although primarily used with couple relationships, it has been used in other relationship contexts.

WHOSE ROLE IS FAMILY WORK?: FAMILY THERAPY VERSUS FAMILY INTERVENTION

At The Oliver Zangwill Centre, it is our view that the responsibility of working with family members belongs to all those working with a client with brain injury. It is important to draw the distinction between "family therapy"—the domain of a small number of qualified family therapists—and "family intervention," which Oddy and Herbert (2003) describe as any interaction between family members and their rehabilitation professionals. Furthermore, this intervention is influenced by therapeutic relationships, the types of challenges being faced, goals, and strategies. Who is involved in delivering the intervention is therefore determined by the team and the client. Figure 10.1 depicts a continuum describing different levels of family intervention.

When intervention is viewed in this way, family therapy or systemic psychotherapy—viewed as a more specialist approach—is at one end of the continuum of interventions, whereas simpler approaches based on educating and sharing information with families are at the other. We would advocate that despite the challenges faced in community settings, such as limited resources, time constraints, and heavy caseloads, it is still possible and necessary to provide family intervention at some level along this continuum. An ideal service model would allow intervention to be provided across the continuum, from developing a shared understanding of brain injury to couple or family therapy. Therapists working in a community setting must determine what level of intervention they or their team can realistically offer to address a family's needs. A referral to external services may be required if the family's needs exceed the team's capacity or capability.

Kreutzer et al. (2010), in their paper on practical approaches to effective family intervention after brain injury, note that establishing and valuing a therapeutic relationship with the client and family is a key aspect. The nature of this relationship significantly determines the outcome of any intervention. A good therapeutic relationship fosters a sense of safety for all, which is essential for the success of interventions. Spending enough time getting to know the person with the injury and the family, and respecting their input into the choice of interventions, will contribute to building an effective therapeutic relationship.

FAMILY INTERVENTION: DEVELOPING A SHARED UNDERSTANDING

Family members of a person with a brain injury often refer to not being consulted or kept informed about their relative's condition and possible treatment. Rolland (1999) states that in order to master the challenges faced in the wake of a chronic disability, family members first need a psychosocial understanding of the condition and its subsequent impact on the family unit; supporting families to achieve this understanding is one of the most basic levels of family intervention. Ideally, this will extend beyond a simple explanation of the mechanics of the injury and its physical consequences to include an appreciation of the experience of living with brain injury for both the individual and the relatives. This type of shared understanding facilitates the type of therapeutic relationship that not only enables the rehabilitation process, but also underpins being able to provide emotional support to the whole family.

The continuum in Figure 10.1 indicates that a shared understanding can be developed through provision of information at a most basic level, but this information must be backed up with constant communication with the family members and collaboration to find ways of meeting their needs.

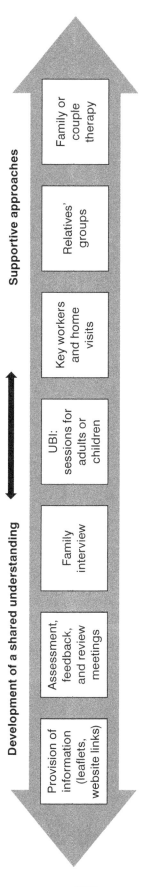

FIGURE 10.1. Continuum describing different levels of family intervention.

Providing Informational Leaflets and Website Links

Leaflets are easy and accessible ways of providing information. Often the timing is not right for a more overt intervention, but family members can keep leaflets to peruse in their own time and at their own pace. This may not take place immediately, but at a time when each family member feels ready, so it is important to have an open policy on where further information can be sought if requested. Many leaflets and other informational documents can be obtained from organizations such as the Brain Injury Association of America (*www.biausa. org*), Headway (*www.headway.org.uk*), the Encephalitis Society (*www.encephalitis.info*), or the Stroke Association (*www.stroke.org.uk*). Websites such as the ones just mentioned and others (e.g., *http://encephalitisglobal.org*, *www.strokeassociation.org*, and *www.brainline. org*) are also good sources of information that families can access in the comfort of their own homes. These websites provide a range of articles related to TBI for people with brain injury and their families. Leaflets and websites that direct families to additional sources of support provide another valuable service. Some of the handouts in this book may also be used as informational leaflets or adapted for this purpose as required.

Assessment, Feedback, and Review Meetings

It can be extremely useful for the rehabilitation team or clinician to meet with family members on a regular basis—not only to keep them updated on the client's rehabilitation progress, but to be updated on the client's and family's life outside rehabilitation in a timely manner. Family members value being included in the rehabilitation process and being part of the "home team" for the client. In cases where there are barriers to meeting in person, speaking on the telephone, using email, or using Skype or similar computer applications can help to keep families in touch with the day-to-day happenings in rehabilitation. In the end, the most important aspects of meetings are finding what works for each client and family, and determining how the team can enable the family to stay involved in and updated on the rehabilitation process.

Understanding Brain Injury: Workshops for Adult Family Members

One-to-one or group education sessions or workshops for families of persons with brain injury can be a valuable way of helping relatives to understand the complexity of the injury and its effects on their loved ones, and to start thinking about helpful strategies. A group format offers the benefits of meeting others in a similar position and of providing opportunities for support; working with an individual family allows the client's formulation to be used as a starting point for creating a tailored session addressing the family's specific questions.

The purpose of such a session should be to help family members make sense of what has happened—not only through understanding the injury itself, but also by connecting the injury to the observed consequences. Suggested content for a group dedicated to understanding brain injury is discussed by Grader and Bateman in Chapter 2 of this workbook. In one-to-one sessions, the information can be tailored to addressing the specific consequences for a particular individual and family, and sessions can take place over a period of time rather than in one sitting.

Understanding Brain Injury: Sessions for Children

Adapting the sessions on understanding brain injury for child relatives usually involves a more practical and playful approach; some suggestions are given below.

Anatomy of the Brain

- Various online interactive tools and neuroanatomy apps for use on mobile devices are available—for example, 3D Brain Interactive (*www.brainline.org/multimedia/interactive_brain/the_human_brain.html*). The application is freely available on the *www.brainline.org* website, which is dedicated to topics on TBI.

- Making a brain out of gelatin is an intriguing activity for many children. Brain-shaped gelatin molds can be sourced online. Strawberry laces or red licorice strings can be used to serve as blood vessels, and three meninges can be created from cling film, bubble wrap, and mesh fabric. The activity is extremely practical, and children usually enjoy eating the gelatin and sweets afterwards.

- Making a brain hat (see Figure 10.2) can help children to remember the functions of different parts of the brain. Ellen McHenry offers a free online template (*www.ellenjmchenry.com/homeschool-freedownloads/lifesciences-games/brainhemishpere.php*).

Cognitive Skills

- *Executive functioning.* Mazes are simple ways of explaining the functions of the frontal lobe, and children also enjoy doing them. There are good online resources for printable mazes for different age groups (one is *http://krazydad.com/mazes*). Other activities could include practical exercises that involve planning and organizing—for example, making a sandwich, constructing a puzzle, or planning an outing.

- *Visual memory.* A memory tray game that we call "Kim's game" at The Oliver Zangwill Centre involves showing the children a tray with between 10 and 12 objects (see Figure 10.3). The children get a set period of time to look at all the objects before they are covered. The aim then is to see how many of the objects the children can recall. This is an example of a visual memory task, but it can also be used to demonstrate strategy use.

- *Verbal memory.* A game we call "Trolley Dash" (in the United States, the equivalent would be "Shopping Cart Dash") is a fun verbal memory game that can be played in a group. The first person starts with the phrase "I went shopping, and in my trolley [or cart] I put a . . ." Each subsequent player then repeats the phrase and adds another item.

- *Attention.* A selective attention test by Simons and Chabris (1999) is available on YouTube and is a fun way to demonstrate attention skills. The video shows a group of people passing a basketball to each other. Some are wearing white T-shirts, while the others are wearing black shirts. Ask the group to count how many times the basketball is passed between the players wearing white shirts. They may or may not notice that a person in a gorilla suit passes through the players at some point during the clip!

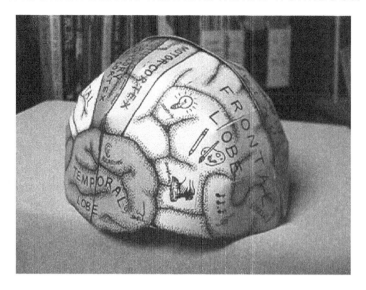

FIGURE 10.2. Brain hat activity. Retrieved from *www.ellenjmchenry.com/ homeschool-freedownloads/lifesciences-games/brainhemishpere.php*   and used by permission of Ellen McHenry.

Visual Processing

A simple exercise is to cover the different quadrants of the lenses in a few pairs of protective goggles and get the children to look at things in this way. The purpose of this exercise is to demonstrate to the children what is it like to view the world with a visual perceptual difficulty—for example, a hemianopia or quadrantanopia.

Language and Communication

   • *Word finding.* Word games like Scrabble are useful ways of demonstrating word finding skills. Sentence construction games, many of which are freely available on the Internet, are fun ways of exploring language processing.

   • *Verbal inhibition/reasoning.* Yes–no games are clever ways of demonstrating verbal inhibition and reasoning. These games involve answering questions asked by others *without* saying yes or no; the children therefore need to think about alternative ways of communicating.

   • *Reading faces.* Difficulty with recognizing emotion through facial expression is a common problem after brain injury. A simple way of demonstrating this skill is to show the group a series of photographs of faces and get the children to identify what emotion is being expressed (e.g., happy, sad, angry, surprised, anxious, or disgusted).

Physical Abilities

   • *Motor cortex.* A fun activity to demonstrate the functions of the motor cortex is to do a dance routine or a circuit of activities. Thinking about which side of the motor cortex is

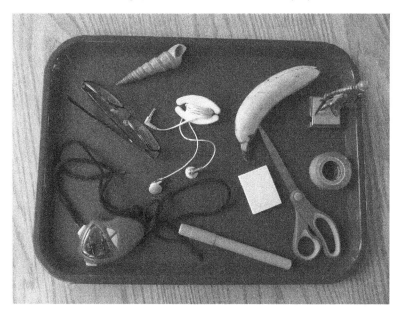

FIGURE 10.3. "Kim's game": A memory tray game.

involved (right or left) while doing an activity, and adding gross and fine motor movements, will help children to understand how the brain controls the body's movements.

• *Sensory cortex.* Place a range of objects with different textures in a large fabric bag or pillowcase. Get each child to feel one object and then guess what it is. Alternatively, blindfold one volunteer; then allow the volunteer to taste a particular flavor (sweet, salty, sour) and to identify the particular taste.

• *Cerebellum.* Set up hopscotch games or other balancing games. If it's possible to obtain a balance board, each child can take a turn trying to balance on the board.

An extensive list of resources, including books, games, and articles, for children of parents with ABI is available from the International Network for Social Workers in Acquired Brain Injury at *www.biswg.co.uk/files/1514/4785/4829/Children-Resource_List_Sept_2012_docx.pdf.*

Providing Support: Key Workers and Home Visits

In a rehabilitation center setting, it can be beneficial for each client's family to be assigned a named "key worker" who liaises with the family on a regular basis throughout rehabilitation, providing a level of support along the way. This role can easily be incorporated into a community setting. Having a person specifically designated as a key worker can ease communication between the team and the family members. Although the nature of the role will differ in every context, it is important to be clear about the boundaries and responsibilities within your individual team. The role may focus on practical issues in some teams, while in others it may consist more of being supportive and offering someone the family members can talk to.

Alongside a family interview, a home visit is another useful way of getting to know the context and the family culture early in the rehabilitation process, especially when the rehabilitation is not being delivered by a domiciliary service. This act of "joining" the family members in their own context also enables a better understanding of the challenges they face, as well as identifying things that might be helpful to rehabilitation in the client's home setting. The complete family context can never be really fully understood even when a worker visits the home, but it is important to check with the family throughout as to how what is done in rehabilitation will fit into family life.

Group Support: Family Days and Relatives' Groups

As noted earlier in this chapter (and as discussed more fully by Gracey et al. in Chapter 9), the impact of the brain injury on an individual's identity is explained in terms of the Y-shaped model, which depicts the felt discrepancy between the preinjury and postinjury selves. Postinjury discrepancy is also experienced by an injured person's family, as differences emerge between the family's identity before and after the injury, and its members struggle to find a new way forward.

One of the ways in which families can be more actively assisted is through forming a relatives' support group. Such a group can be facilitated in a community setting, as well as in a rehabilitation center; it may be of a fixed duration (e.g., a 6-week program) or more open-ended. The purpose of the group is to support relatives in coming to terms with and adjusting to the changing situation. Ideally, a group would be facilitated by a systemic practitioner and a clinical psychologist. In a community setting, there may or may not be professionals with this particular skill set; however, a similar group facilitated by other professionals or paraprofessionals, and focusing on brain injury's consequences and more practical strategies for dealing with these, can provide opportunities for peer support.

The opportunity for members of a client's family to "offload" some of the stress they are experiencing can be most valuable. Feeling validated and able to articulate the difficulties they are experiencing as a family, without being judged by others, can support the family in moving forward. At the same time, the clinicians or other facilitators can gain a better understanding of the lived experience of each family in the group—an understanding that is often missed in the rehabilitation process, as the focus is on the persons with brain injury.

Support groups can also focus on specific approaches. For example, conversational partner work, adapted for ABI from communication work in stroke (Pound, 2004), focuses mainly on the communication between a person with brain injury and a family member and explores ways of communicating that are helpful to the relationship. Other topics might include ways to minimize caregiver strain, sources of practical or emotional support for family members, and sharing of useful strategies.

The idea of "outsider witnessing," taken from narrative therapy, can be used in the community just as well as in rehabilitation centers. An adapted version of the approach involves inviting past clients and/or family members to talk to a group about their experience. Often meeting someone who has been in a similar situation is very valuable, especially when they are further along in the journey through rehabilitation.

It goes without saying that it is important to consider group rules, confidentiality, and boundaries, in order to protect the family members and clients; to discuss these issues openly with the group; and to repeat this process regularly.

Referral to More Intensive Services

Finally, support can sometimes take the form of determining that a family's needs are beyond the scope of what your rehabilitation service can provide. This can involve referral to family or couple therapy services, counseling services, or caregiver support organizations. Having regular ongoing contact with a client's family puts a clinician in a good position to notice when the caregiver or family might need more support. The therapeutic relationship that has been developed can facilitate a smooth handover to other specialist services.

REFERENCES

Ben-Yishay, Y. (2000). Post acute neuropsychological rehabilitation: A holistic perspective. In A. L. Christensen & B. P. Uzzell (Eds.), *International handbook of neuropsychological rehabilitation* (pp. 127–135). New York: Kluwer Academic/Plenum.

Bowen, C. (2007). Family therapy and neurorehabilitation: Forging a link. *International Journal of Therapy and Rehabilitation, 14*(8), 344–349.

Bowen, C., Yeates, G., & Palmer, S. (2010). *A relational approach to rehabilitation: Thinking about relationships after brain injury.* London: Karnac.

Brooks, D. N. (1991). The head-injured family. *Journal of Clinical and Experimental Neuropsychology, 13*, 155–188.

Burnham, J. (1986). Transitions. In J. B. Burnham, *Family therapy: First steps towards a systemic approach* (pp. 25–44). London: Routledge.

Butcher, J. (2006). *Proven guilty.* New York: Penguin.

Dallos, R., & Draper, R. (2010). *An introduction to family therapy: Systemic theory and practice.* Maidenhead, UK: Open University Press.

DePompei, R., & Williams, J. (1994). Working with families after TBI: A family-centred approach. *Topics in Language Disorders, 15*(1), 68–81.

Hall, K. M., Karzmak, P., Stevens, M., Englander, J., O'Hare, P., & Wright, J. (1994). Family stressors in traumatic brain injury: A two-year follow-up. *Archives of Physical Medicine and Rehabilitation, 75*, 876–884.

Hsu, N., Kreutzer, J., & Menzel, J. (2009, June). Family change after brain injury. Retrieved from *http://brainline.org/content/2009/06/family-change-after-brain-injury.html*

Johnson, J. L., & McCown, W. G. (1997). *Family therapy of neurobehavioral disorders: Integrating neuropsychology and family therapy.* New York: Haworth Press.

Knight, R. G., Deveraux, R., & Godfrey, H. P. (1998). Caring for a family member with a traumatic brain injury. *Brain Injury, 12*(6), 467–481.

Kreutzer, J. S., Marwitz, J. H., Godwin, E. E., & Arango-Lasprilla, J. C. (2010). Practical approaches to effective family intervention after brain injury. *Journal of Head Trauma Rehabilitation, 25*(2), 113–120.

Langlois, J. A., Rutland-Brown, W., & Wald, M. M. (2006). The epidemiology and impact of traumatic brain injury: A brief overview. *Journal of Head Trauma Rehabilitation, 21*, 375–378.

Leber, W. R., & Jenkins, M. R. (1996). Psychotherapy with clients who have brain injuries and their families. In L. Russell (Ed.), *Neuropsychology for clinical practice: Etiology, assessment and treatment* (pp. 489–505). Washington, DC: American Psychological Association.

Lehan, T., Arango-Lasprilla, J. C., de los Reyes, C. J., & Quijano, M. C. (2012). The ties that bind: The relationship between caregiver burden and the neuropsychological functioning of TBI survivors. *NeuroRehabilitation, 30*(1), 87–95.

Lezak, M. (1988). Brain damage is a family affair. *Journal of Clinical and Experimental Neuropsychology, 10*(1), 111–123.

Oddy, M., & Herbert, C. (2003). Interventions with families following brain injury: Evidence-based practice. *Neuropsychological Rehabilitation, 13*(1–2), 259–273.

Pound, C. (2004). Dare to be different: The person and the practice. In J. F. Duchan & S. Byng (Eds.), *Challenging aphasia therapies: Broadening the discourse and extending the boundaries* (pp. 32–53). Hove, UK: Psychology Press.

Rolland, J. S. (1999). Parental illness and disability: A family systems framework. *Journal of Family Therapy, 21,* 242–266.

Simons, D. J., & Chabris, C. F. (1999). Gorillas in our midst: Sustained inattentional blindness for dynamic events. *Perception, 28*(9), 1059–1074.

Spanier, G. B. (1976). Measuring dyadic adjustment: New scales for assessing the quality of marriage and similar dyads. *Journal of Marriage and the Family, 38,* 15–28.

Spanier, G. B. (1989). *Manual for the Dyadic Adjustment Scale.* North Tonawanda, NY: Multi-Health Systems.

Wilson, B. A., Gracey, F., Malley, D., Evans, J. J., & Bateman, A. (2009). The Oliver Zangwill Centre approach to neuropsychological rehabilitation. In B. A. Wilson, F. Gracey, J. J. Evans, & A. Bateman, *Neuropsychological rehabilitation: Theory, models, therapy and outcome* (pp. 47–67). Cambridge, UK: Cambridge University Press.

Yeates, G. (2009). Working with families in neuropsychological rehabilitation. In B. A. Wilson, F. Gracey, J. J. Evans, & A. Bateman (Eds.), *Neuropsychological rehabilitation: Theory, models, therapy and outcomes* (pp. 138–156). Cambridge, UK: Cambridge University Press.

Index

Note: The letter *f* after a page number indicates figure; *t* indicates table; and *h* indicates handout.